Winning with Osteoporosis

Other books by Drs. McIlwain, Silverfield, and Burnette
and Debra Fulghum Bruce:

Winning with Arthritis
Winning with Back Pain
The 50+ Wellness Program

Winning with Osteoporosis

Harris H. McIlwain, MD
Debra Fulghum Bruce
Joel C. Silverfield, MD
Michael C. Burnette, MD
Bernard F. Germain, MD

John Wiley & Sons, Inc.
New York • Chichester • Brisbane • Toronto • Singapore

To those who wish to know
that prevention and treatment of
osteoporosis are possible,
and to Linda and Bob,
whose support and encouragement
have been unending.

This text is printed on acid-free paper.

Copyright © 1993 by John Wiley & Sons, Inc.

All rights reserved. Published simultaneously in Canada.

Reproduction or translation of any part of this work beyond
that permitted by Section 107 or 108 of the 1976 United
States Copyright Act without the permission of the copyright
owner is unlawful. Requests for permission or further
information should be addressed to the Permissions Department,
John Wiley & Sons, Inc., 605 Third Avenue, New York, NY
10158-0012.

This publication is designed to provide accurate and
authoritative information in regard to the subject
matter covered. It is sold with the understanding that
the publisher is not engaged in rendering legal, accounting,
or other professional services. If legal advice or other
expert assistance is required, the services of a competent
professional person should be sought. *From a Declaration
of Principles jointly adopted by a Committee of the
American Bar Association and a Committee of Publishers.*

Library of Congress Cataloging in Publication Data:

Osteoporosis.
    Winning with osteoporosis / Harris H. McIlwain . . . [et al.]. —
[2nd ed.]
        p. cm.
    Previous ed. published under the title: Osteoporosis.
    Includes bibliographical references and index.
    ISBN 0-471-30489-1 (acid-free paper : pbk.)
    1. Osteoporosis—Popular works. 2. Osteoporosis—Prevention.
I. McIlwain, Harris H. II. Title.
RC931.0730776 1994
616.7'16—dc20   93-7530

Printed in the United States of America

10 9 8 7 6 5 4 3 2 1

Preface

"Painfully expensive," that's how one patient described her recent nine-day stay in the hospital after a hip fracture. Painful, because the fractured hip caused by osteoporosis made it difficult to even sit up much less be mobile, and expensive, because the lengthy stay cost her and the insurance company over $30,000.

As our nation tries to control the skyrocketing costs of personal health care, we are looking for ways to lessen the need for expensive hospital stays due to injury. Now it may be possible to prevent injuries such as these fractures from occurring in the first place.

Osteoporosis is a savage disease that results in painful and debilitating fractures. As the disease progresses, bones become thin and break easily. Although osteoporosis affects over 30 million Americans, it can now be prevented and even successfully treated. The fractures that once caused severe pain and expensive hospital stays may now be controlled.

No cure is known yet, but there are ways to tell if you are at risk for osteoporosis years before the disease is evident. Understanding osteoporosis will allow you to begin the process of prevention. If osteoporosis is already present, early detection is available, allowing treatment. This treatment does work and can greatly improve your future by delaying or halting the disease. You *can* make a difference.

The facts seem frightening.

- 20 percent of persons with hip fractures may need a nursing home or other facility for up to one year.
- 20 percent may not walk the first year.
- Up to 50 percent may never walk as well as they did before the fracture.
- 20 percent may die within the first year because of multiple medical problems.

Each of these outcomes involves a great human cost that makes prevention and treatment of osteoporosis a worthwhile goal. The financial burden for this disease is high. In the United States, fractures cost over $10 billion per year, with the direct costs of hip fractures greater than $7 billion! There are also many indirect costs, including nursing home care and loss of the ability to do daily activities.

Osteoporosis is the main culprit causing over 80 percent of these hip fractures. If some percentage of these hip fractures could be prevented, the savings would be great in medical costs and suffering. If we do not take some action, it is likely that medical expenses due to osteoporosis will continue to soar.

Who is at risk? Although osteoporosis can occur in anyone, the risk of the disease and the resulting fractures is highest in those over age 65. Because our population is living longer, there will be more people at risk as time progresses. By the turn of the century, it is estimated that over 50 million Americans will be age 65 or older. One person out of six will be over the age of 65—about double today's numbers. If we do not lower the number of hip fractures, the direct cost of this problem alone may exceed $20 billion each year. The total costs would be even higher.

Education about osteoporosis prevention and treatment is the first step toward lowering the cost of fractures and health care. Knowledge of risk factors, a plan for prevention, and the latest methods of treatment can significantly lower our total health care bill.

Winning with Osteoporosis gives the latest facts and shows you the steps you can take to understand:

- What osteoporosis is.
- Who it affects.
- How to tell if you are at risk.
- How to tell if you might have the disease.
- What steps are necessary for prevention.
- What the best available treatments are.

No one course of treatment is the answer for everyone. While the treatments suggested in this book will not cure osteoporosis, they will help to relieve your pain or discomfort, maintain or increase your mobility, and halt bone loss before it is too late.

Finally, this book is not a substitute for medical care. After reading this book, talk with your physician, and choose a personal program that will satisfy you and enable you to begin managing your osteoporosis.

Acknowledgments

We would like to make special note of the work of the many people who made this book possible: Francis I. Barford, L.O.T.R.; Arthur Frommor, Travel Editor; Roy E. Fulghum; Susan Haley, R.D.; Dorothy P. Judson; Mary A. Sprinkle, R.D.; Lori F. Steinmeyer, M.S., R.D., L.D.; Vicki K. Winsor, R.P.T.

To all of these talented individuals, we give our deepest appreciation.

TRADEMARKS

Advil is a trademark of Whitehall Laboratories, Inc.
Alkamints is a trademark of Miles Inc. Consumer Healthcare Division.
Anacin is a trademark of Whitehall Laboratories, Inc.
Arby's is a trademark of Arby's, Inc.
Aristocort is a trademark of Lederle Laboratories; a division of American Cyanimid Company.
Aygestin is a trademark of Ayerst Laboratories Division of American Home Products Corporation.
Banquet is a trademark of Conagra Frozen Foods.
Big Mac is a trademark of McDonalds.
Biocal is a trademark of Miles, Inc., Consumer Healthcare Division.
Breakfast Croissan'wich is a trademark of Burger King.
Buster Bar is a trademark of International Dairy Queen.
Calciferol is a trademark of Kremers-Urban Company.
Calcimar is a trademark of USV Laboratories Division of USV Pharmaceuticals Corp.
Calcet is a trademark of Mission Pharmaceutical Company.
Cal-Sup is a trademark of 3M Corporation.
Campbells is a trademark of the Campbell Soup Company.
Celeste is a trademark of the Quaker Oats Company.
Celestone is a trademark of Schering Corporation.
Danny in a Cup is a trademark of the Dannon Company, Inc.
Darvon is a trademark of Eli Lilly and Company.
Decadron is a trademark of Merck Sharp & Dohme Division of Merck & Co., Inc.
Del Monte is a trademark of the Del Monte Corporation.
Dical-D is a trademark of Abbott Laboratories Pharmaceutical Products Division.
Dilly Bar is a trademark of International Dairy Queen.
Dorcol is a trademark of Sandoz Consumer Health Care Group Division of Sandoz, Inc.
Egg McMuffin is a trademark of McDonalds.
Estrace is a trademark of Mead Johnson, Bristol-Myers, U.S. Pharmaceuticals, and Nutritional Group.
Estraderm is a trademark of Ciba Pharmaceutical Company Division of Ciba-Geigy Corporation.
Estratab is a trademark of Reid-Rowell.
Estrovis is a trademark of Parke-David Division of Warner-Lambert Company.
French Toast Sticks is a trademark of Burger King.
Franco American is a trademark of the Campbell Soup Company.
Great Danish is a trademark of Burger King.
Heinz is a trademark of the H. J. Heinz Company.
Lactaid is a trademark of Lactaid Inc.
Medipren is a trademark of McNeil Consumer Products Company.
Medrol is a trademark of Upjohn Company.
Mr. Misty is a trademark of International Dairy Queen.
Neo-Glucagon is a trademark of Sandoz Consumer Health Care Group Division of Sandoz, Inc.
Nuprin is a trademark of Bristol-Meyers Products Division of Bristol-Meyers Co.
Ogen is a trademark of Abbott Laboratories, Pharmaceuticals Products Division.
Pizza Hut is a trademark of Pizza Hut of America, Inc.
Premarin is a trademark of Ayerst Laboratories; Division of American Home Products Corporation.
Sealtest is a trademark of Kraft, Inc.
Swanson is a trademark of the Campbell Soup Company.
Taco Bell is a trademark of the Taco Bell Corporation.
Titralac is a trademark of 3M Corporation.
Tylenol is a trademark of McNeil Consumer Products Company.
Wendy's is a trademark of Wendy's International, Inc.
Whaler is a trademark of Burger King.
Whopper is a trademark of Burger King.
Yoplait is a trademark of Yoplait, USA, Inc.

Contents

Introduction:
What Is Osteoporosis?

When a 63-year-old patient was told that according to a bone density test she had lost 35 percent of the bone in her hip, she was shocked. "Losing bone? How is that possible?" she asked with concern.

The truth is that our bodies are constantly building new bone and removing old bone. In younger people, more bone is built than is removed resulting in growth of bones and an increase in the total amount. After maturity is reached at age 30 to 40, the amount of bone removed gradually becomes greater than the amount of bone formed. As a result, the total amount of bone decreases.

Osteoporosis results from this gradual decrease in the amount of bone present in our bodies. By age 60, it is common for a woman to have lost 20 percent or more of the bone present in her body in earlier years. Some conditions make the bone loss occur earlier or more rapidly. In fact, this bone loss is so common that it is usually thought of as "normal" in the process of aging. This bone loss *should not be accepted* as normal or necessary, just as fractures should not be considered a normal part of aging.

If the bone loss continues, over a number of years enough bone will be lost so that the bones are weakened, breaking easily. With all of the advances in modern medicine, women and men are living longer lives. This means more years in which the gradual loss of bone continues. Eventually, enough bone is lost so that fractures happen when minor injuries occur. After many years, even normal stress on bones such as sitting, standing, or minor stress such as bending or lifting, can cause a fracture. After more and more fractures, there may be constant severe pain, deformity, and crippling.

Twenty-five percent of women over age 60 have fractures in the spine from osteoporosis. Up to 40 percent have some fracture after age 65. A fracture of the spine happens when one of the spine's vertebral bones loses height, and usually appears on X-ray to be compressed (Figure 1). By age 75, 50 percent of all women have compression in the spine.

If osteoporosis could be prevented or treated in these people, consider the savings possible in pain, suffering, and expense! In fact, prevention and treatment *are possible* for osteoporosis.

Osteoporosis can be divided into 4 stages—from Stage 1 when osteoporosis is not even detectable to Stage 4 with chronic fractures and deformity. See Table 1 for a review of the course of the stages of osteoporosis and corresponding symptoms. As

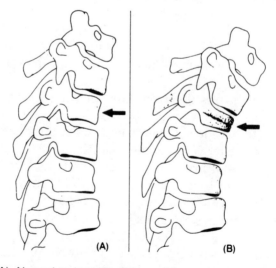

Figure 1. (A) Normal spine (B) Spine with compression fracture. Note shortening of vertebra and abnormal curve of spine.

TABLE 1
The Course of Osteoporosis

Stage	Begins	
Stage 1	Begins sometime after reaching young adult age (Age 30-40)	Before osteoporosis is detectable
Stage 2	Age 35-55	Osteoporosis becomes detectable
Stage 3	Age 45 and older	Osteoporosis results in fracture of bones
Stage 4	Age 55 and older	Osteoporosis with chronic pain and deformity

you understand which stage in the development of osteoporosis best fits your situation, the guidelines for prevention and treatment become easier to understand and follow. This allows you to be sure that you are receiving the best possible treatment available. (See Figure 2.)

Stage 1 is the period before osteoporosis becomes detectable. At some point after we reach the age of a young adult, there is a gradual decrease in the total amount or density of bone in the body. This loss is gradual and is not yet possible to detect for a number of years. During this time, the body is constantly building and removing bone. The balance of the two processes slowly shifts so that gradually more bone is removed than is formed. The bones are still strong, exhibiting no pain and no unusual fractures. The greater the amount of bone present at the beginning of this stage (the denser the bones), the longer the density of the bones will last.

If we could somehow detect the start of this process and begin treatment, it is likely that the outcome would be much more positive than it is today. During this time, the disease is silent and there is absolutely no way for you to tell by the way you feel or by the most thorough examination that this process is happening. Until such a test becomes available, there are good clues to predict which people are at high risk for the later development of osteoporosis. If you have one or more of the risk factors outlined in Chapter Three, then following the guidelines for prevention may delay or prevent the occurrence

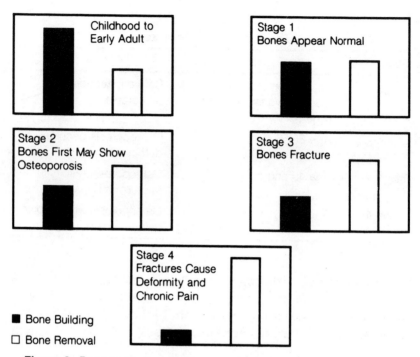

Figure 2. Bar graphs showing the course of osteoporosis in 4 stages.

of osteoporosis many years later. Unfortunately, Stage 1 is the stage when prevention is most effective, but the problem is least noticeable.

Stage 2 usually begins sometime after age 35. The very gradual loss of bone has continued for a number of years, but the remaining bone is still strong enough so that unusual fractures do not happen. Of course, with severe injuries fractures can occur, but there are still no fractures following minor injury. Activities that have been done over many years can still be performed. Unless you know that you are at a higher level of risk, there is still no sign or feeling to let you know of osteoporosis or future fractures. But in this stage, the osteoporosis first becomes detectable by testing. Routine X-rays may show a compression fracture of the spine or decreased density of some bone. The problem is that before X-rays are able to detect osteoporosis, about 30 percent of the bone has already been lost! X-rays are not a very good way to detect osteoporosis early.

There are tests available that can detect osteoporosis at the earliest possible stage. It is still hard to predict whether there will actually be fractures and when the fractures might happen. But the tests can accurately tell how much (if any) osteoporosis is present. Best of all, these tests can find osteoporosis *years* before fractures happen. Then treatment can begin to strengthen the bones and prevent fractures. And treatment works! Chapter Four explains the tests.

Stage 3—osteoporosis with bone fractures—often begins around age 55 or older, but can happen earlier if more than 1 or 2 risk factors are present. As you can now tell, the osteoporosis process has been present for many years. At Stage 3, the bones become thin enough so that injuries (which before this stage were not noticed) now cause a fracture of a bone. This is most common in the spine, especially in the lower back or lumbar spine, in the hips, and in the wrists. The basic problem is that enough bone has been lost to cause weakening of the remaining bone. A minor fall or injury results in fracture. This is the stage when the bone in a hip may break from osteoporosis. The person may fall *because* the hip breaks. This is often overlooked—it is assumed that the person fell first!

We saw a 55-year-old woman who is active, independent, and manages her own large business. She had been healthy with no limitations until 10 months earlier. At that time, she had a minor fall when she tripped over a 1-inch change in the level of the sidewalk. From that time, she had severe back pain. It was found on X-ray that she had severe osteoporosis and two fractures of the spinal vertebrae. The osteoporosis had been present for many years! Had she known this years earlier she may well have prevented this problem.

Other areas can be affected by fractures in Stage 3. Any bone may be involved, including feet, ankles, shoulders, wrists, and pelvis. If the osteoporosis is found as a result of the fracture, treatment can be started. Then, hopefully, more crippling fractures can be prevented.

If the process of osteoporosis continues, the bones become thinner each year. Stage 4 may begin after age 55 years, or can happen earlier if many risk factors are present. In Stage 4, more fractures occur, usually with more and more pain. The most common areas affected are still the spine, especially the middle and lower back areas called the thoracic and lumbar spine. Since each fracture of a vertebrae in the spine causes it to become a little shorter, as more fractures occur, the person experiences loss of height.

This is one of the reasons older people often lose height. It has been estimated that a compression fracture in one of the spinal vertebrae causes an average loss of height of about 0.5 cm or $1/4$ inch (Figure 3).

It is easy to see why, after a few years, several inches in height may be lost.

In addition, the shape of the spine may change. The fractures often cause the vertebral body, which is normally square, to become more wedge-shaped as it compresses because of the forces of the weight of the body (see Figure 1, p. 2).

This results in the familiar "dowager's hump" and eventually in a stooped appearance. This is actually the end result of many years of osteoporosis. The picture usually shown of a lady with osteoporosis with a stooped look is therefore a late stage of osteoporosis (Figure 4).

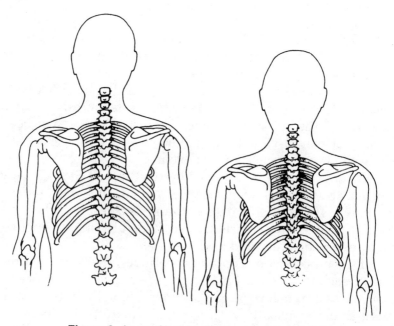

Figure 3. Loss of height due to spinal shortening.

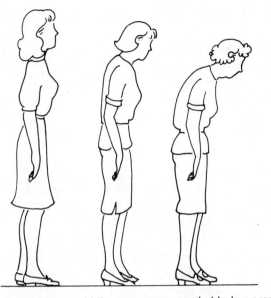

Figure 4. A young woman, middle-age woman, and elderly woman showing bending of spine and loss of height due to osteoporosis.

Fractures of the hip are very common. This fracture actually refers to several different kinds of fractures, usually in the upper part of the large bone in the thigh, the femur (Figure 5).

The actual fracture can happen at one of several parts of the bone. The severe results of fractures of the hip were discussed earlier.

Fractures may happen in the pelvic bones after a fall and result in severe pain in the lower abdomen, pelvic area, and

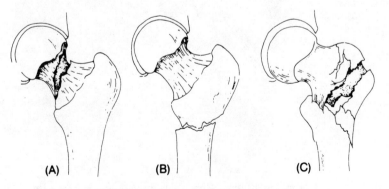

(A) (B) (C)

Figure 5. Three of the most common types of hip fracture.

groin. This usually requires days or weeks in bed or in the hospital.

As this stage becomes more severe, less common fractures begin to happen. We recently saw a patient who suffered a broken rib after coughing! One lady had severe osteoporosis as a result of being 62 years old, having severe arthritis, and being treated for many years with cortisone. She recently had hospital stays for fractures in both hips that required surgery. She had lost 3 inches in height due to vertebrae fractures.

As you might expect, after several fractures, in addition to deformity, pain becomes constant and severe. The pain is usually concentrated in the middle and lower back. Gradually this constant pain becomes a major problem. Walking becomes more and more difficult due to the back pain and the stooped posture. The ribs move closer to the pelvic bones as the spine becomes more curved (Figure 6). The back deformity may make the abdomen appear pushed forward and be painful.

Pain medications, even narcotics, do not usually give much relief. Stage 4 is very difficult for the patient and the physician. But even then there is treatment available to help prevent future fractures and minimize pain.

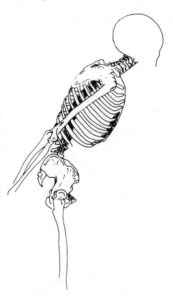

Figure 6. The dowager's hump. Note that the lowest ribs almost touch the pelvis bone.

What Causes Osteoporosis?

There is no single cause of osteoporosis. In most people affected, there are many factors that contribute to the disease. Some people are much more likely to develop osteoporosis than others. This higher risk can be predicted in many people if risk factors for osteoporosis are known. These are discussed in Chapter Two.

For example, being a cigarette smoker, underweight, and having a low-calcium diet all seem to be common factors in many osteoporosis patients. These risk factors are often treatable, but they must be detected early. If people who are at risk for osteoporosis are identified early, proper treatment may delay or prevent the development of the problem. Then the chance of broken bones, loss of height, and crippling also declines.

The female hormone system, especially estrogen, is important in bone formation. As the amount of estrogen in the body decreases at menopause, more bone is lost, less bone is formed, and the bones often become thinner. If menopause happens early, osteoporosis can begin early.

There are inherited or genetic factors. For example, white women seem most at risk for osteoporosis, with less risk for white men. African-American women have much less osteoporosis and fewer fractures than white women, and African-American men seem to have even lower amounts of osteoporosis and fractures. The exact reasons for these variations are not known.

Other problems may increase the risk of osteoporosis. Thin people have more osteoporosis than overweight people. Heavy alcohol use and cigarette smoking seem to increase the chance of osteoporosis as well.

Activity, especially weight-bearing activity, definitely stimulates new bone formation. This has been shown in animals. It has been known for years that patients immobilized by bedrest and even healthy astronauts on weightless space flights develop thinner bones. Athletes generally have stronger bones than nonathletes, but excessive training in women may actually cause more osteoporosis.

It has been found that women who engage in severe physical training such as prolonged, long-distance running may develop less regular menstrual periods. The menstrual periods may even stop temporarily, as a result of changes in estrogen levels due to physical training. These changes in hormone levels in some cases can result in loss of bone mass, osteoporosis, and fractures.

Other causes of osteoporosis will be discussed in this book. Some illnesses can increase the chance of osteoporosis.

None of the current theories completely explain the disease osteoporosis. Future research will come closer to defining the causes of osteoporosis and will, hopefully, allow better treatment to be developed.

If you learn what the risk factors are, you can begin to treat and correct the problems. Decide which stage fits your situation best and follow the guidelines outlined in Chapters Four and Five for prevention and treatment of osteoporosis. The earlier the risk factors are found and other medical problems corrected, the better the prevention. If osteoporosis is already present, you can begin treatment that works. Bones can become stronger to lower the chance of fractures in the future.

SUMMARY

1. Our bodies constantly build and remove bone.
2. After young adulthood, there is a gradual decrease in the amount of bone present.
3. Stages in the course of osteoporosis:
   STAGE 1: Gradual bone loss begins, but is not detectable (ages 30 and over).
   STAGE 2: Enough bone loss has happened to become detectable (ages 35–55).
   STAGE 3: More bone loss; fractures happen more easily (ages 45 and over).
   STAGE 4: More fractures, deformity, crippling, and constant pain (ages 55 and over).
4. There are clues to predict which people are at high risk for osteoporosis. These are discussed in Chapter Three.

CHAPTER ONE

You *Can* Win
with Osteoporosis

You have heard the story before . . . a person falls and suffers a broken hip. An operation is needed in order for the person to walk again. Many times this happens to a person who is already burdened with other illnesses. The broken hip may cause complications that could result in more serious illnesses—even death.

As many as 20 percent of such patients may not walk after one year, and as many as 20 percent of such patients may die within one year of a hip fracture. As mentioned earlier, the cost of hip fracture alone in this country is estimated to be $7 billion each year.

Osteoporosis is the basic cause of this problem and affects over 30 million people in America. While this painful disease begins gradually and silently, by age 65, as many as 80 percent of women in our population may have osteoporosis and 25 percent may have fractures. The statistics are high. Over 30 million people, the majority of whom are women, are affected by osteoporosis. The frightening fact is that most people who have osteoporosis are undiagnosed. Yet, the good news is that almost everyone with osteoporosis can be treated.

The next few pages could change your life. The facts, current research reports, and other timely information will change your attitude toward this disease.

If you have osteoporosis, this book will offer important suggestions on how you can manage the disease and live a normal, active life while limiting the debilitating pain associated with it. If you have not been diagnosed as having osteoporosis, this book can give you important information to help prevent the disease. The explanations of the four stages of osteoporosis, the signs and symptoms of the disease, and the plan for prevention and treatment can guide you to a healthier, fuller life.

Osteoporosis: Thinning of the Bones

Osteoporosis means a decrease in the density of the bone, or more simply put, thinning of the bones. As bones become thinner, they become easier to break. Usual daily activities such as standing, walking, and bending may be enough to cause a broken bone. These fractures can occur in the back, the hip, the foot, or other bones. Minor injuries that usually go unnoticed result in a fracture with severe pain, limitation, and expense. It is estimated that in the United States over 1.5 million fractures happen each year due to osteoporosis. This results in disability, hospitalization, and a cost of over $10 billion annually.

Case Studies

A 58-year-old woman was seen in our clinic. She had fallen at home in the bathtub and had severe hip pain. She was found to have a fracture of the hip (femur) and required a hospital stay of 10 days with an operation to allow the hip to heal properly (see Figure 5, p. 7). The hospital bill was over $30,000. Common complications that can happen in this situation, even with the best care, include blood clot formation, bleeding, infection, and other medical problems. Each of these complications could result in a much more serious illness, prolonged hospital stay, and even death.

We saw another patient recently. This 62-year-old woman had been very active in many activities, especially golf. She tripped while walking to her car and suffered a severe fracture of the ankle and foot. This one fracture required surgery and forced her to be off her feet for six weeks. Her hospital bill was over $8,000. She required four months to resume her usual activity. This woman was found to have osteoporosis and began treatment including calcium, vitamin D, and other medications. Had she known about her osteoporosis years earlier, she may have prevented this unfortunate accident.

Over 30 Million Sufferers

Although over 30 million people are affected by osteoporosis, this painful disease is more common in women, especially after menopause. We saw a 60-year-old lady who had no fractures, but who was concerned about osteoporosis because her mother died after a hip fracture. She is white, had menopause 10 years ago, and never took estrogen treatment. On bone density testing she was found to have osteoporosis, in fact, was found to have bone density about 30 percent below normal.

She began to remove risk factors, started an exercise program, began estrogen treatment, and took calcium supplements. After one year, her bone density increased slightly without other medications. By repeating her bone density test in one to two years, she will know if further bone loss occurs. She can add other effective medications, accordingly.

A 62-year-old lady was seen who had broken a rib in a minor fall and was concerned about osteoporosis. She had several family members who suffered from the disease. She had gone through menopause at age 48 and had not taken estrogen. With simple testing, she was found to have a loss of about 35 percent of the bone in her lower (lumbar) spine.

She began calcium, exercises, and a walking program, and was given estrogen and other medications. After two years, repeat tests showed an increase in bone density of 9 percent in her spine. Along with this increase in bone density, her risk of future fractures became less. Hopefully her improvement will continue.

We now know that there is a gradual decrease in the amount of bone after the age of 30 to 40 years that happens more rapidly in women than in men. By the age of about 65 years, most women have a significant problem with osteoporosis. Let us emphasize again that statistics report as many as 80 percent of women over 65 years old have osteoporosis and 25 percent of women over 65 may have fractures.

It has been found that up to 20 percent of women in their 40s may be affected by osteoporosis. Men are also affected although fractures seem to happen later in life for men than in women. There is no magic way for you to know whether you have osteoporosis and how mild or severe it may be.

If the disease goes undetected and untreated, you could be at a high risk for a fracture. Unfortunately, the bones that are most commonly fractured are those important in allowing you to remain active—the hip and back, especially the lower part of the back or lumbar spine (Figure 7). Over time, your back may become bent or stooped, you may lose inches in height, and you may suffer severe constant pain when you stand or walk.

More and more often we see women who know about osteoporosis and fractures. Another woman was seen who was 71 and remains a very active traveler, including frequent international travel. She had severe back pain and was found to have osteoporosis and a fracture in the lower spine.

She began an exercise program, calcium, and vitamin D supplements, along with other medications. Within 10 months, her bone density test showed an increase of over 3 percent. Since she may have been losing bone each year, this was excellent improvement in a relatively short time.

Types of Osteoporosis

Current researchers divide osteoporosis into 2 types, but these are not always clearly defined and mixtures are common.

One type of osteoporosis, according to some researchers, is most common in women after menopause. This typically occurs after age 50. Fractures are most common in the spine (vertebral fractures) and in the wrists. It is thought that the lower level of estrogen after menopause is the basic problem and causes more rapid removal of the bone. The intestine also

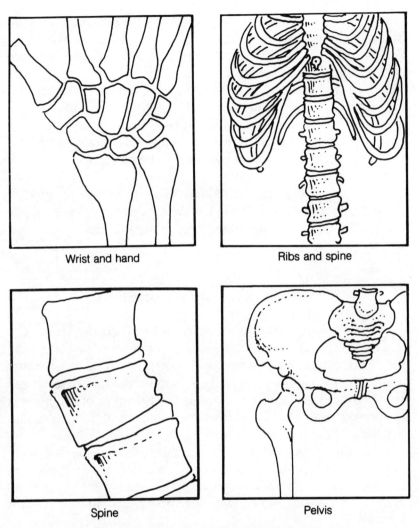

Wrist and hand

Ribs and spine

Spine

Pelvis

Figure 7. Bones most frequently fractured.

seems less able to absorb the calcium which is necessary for bone formation. As a result, more bone is removed and less bone is formed.

Another type of osteoporosis occurs in men and women at an older age, usually 70 to 75 years of age. The most common area of fracture is the hip. As people age, it is thought that less vitamin D is produced by the body. Vitamin D is necessary for calcium absorption from the intestine. Again, when the intestine is less able to absorb calcium, less bone is formed while bone removal continues.

Another theory is that the process of bone building and removal are normally "coupled" at the correct rates. This process for some reason becomes "uncoupled," and bone formation slows down but bone removal continues. Or, bone removal increases but the rate of bone building does not. The causes of "uncoupling" are not known.

Although other problems may raise the risk of osteoporosis, little is understood about the actual reasons. However, the earlier the problems are recognized and corrected, the better the results.

Detecting Osteoporosis

Usually you do not find out that you have osteoporosis until a bone is broken. At this time, an X-ray is taken, and the fracture and osteoporosis are diagnosed (Figure 8). With more awareness of osteoporosis and its symptoms, this disease can be discovered at an earlier time. If the thinning of the bone is overlooked, only the actual fracture will be treated, resulting in further fractures and disability.

If you think you may be at risk for osteoporosis, what can be done? First, talk with your physician. A simple test can tell how much (if any) osteoporosis you have. This test can give you an indication of whether you are at a higher risk for fracture.

Once a diagnosis of osteoporosis is made, it is important to look for any other diseases that might be contributing so proper treatment can be given for these separate problems.

After the condition is diagnosed, the available treatment should start immediately, including supplements to strengthen bones and medications, if needed, to slow the removal of bone.

These treatments help the body build stronger and more bone tissue and can reduce the risk of fractures. If the number of hip fractures could be reduced, there would be great savings

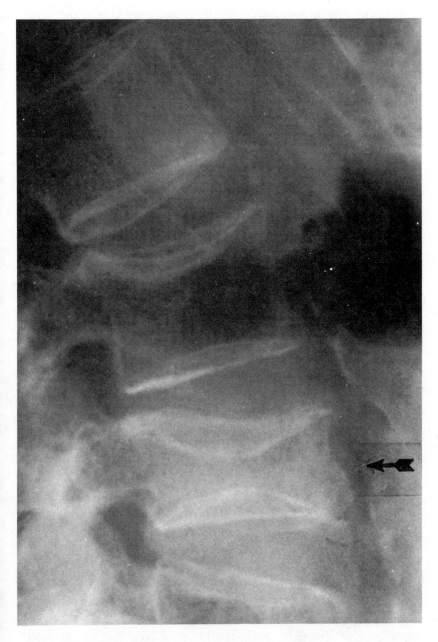

Figure 8. The arrow shows a bone in the spine shorter than the others because of a fracture.

in hospital costs, pain, and suffering. If spine fractures could be reduced or prevented, the severe pain and deformity of the spine could be better controlled.

Managing Your Osteoporosis

We now know more about the prevention of osteoporosis, which is best begun at the earliest possible time. In most people, this means starting prevention even in childhood, before bone thinning is present. There is new hope for osteoporosis victims as new and better treatments become available. With proper diagnosis and a specific plan of treatment, you can slow the progress of the thinning bones and can actually restore stronger bone development.

In successfully managing your osteoporosis, it is important that you become aware of the kinds of treatment available. You must know which treatments are likely to be effective, which treatments will probably not work well, and take immediate steps in choosing the correct treatment for you. You can greatly help your physician in the management of your problem if you know the guidelines suggested in this book.

In our clinic, osteoporosis patients ask questions such as:

Q: Will I have to limit my activity with this disease?

Q: Since there is pain involved, should I force myself in spite of the pain?

Q: Does my diet affect my disease?

Q: What are some of the other important ways to manage osteoporosis?

Q: Does the pain ever improve, or must I live with it forever?

It turns out there are no absolute or magic answers to these questions. However, with an accurate understanding of what happens in osteoporosis and what treatments are available, you can create a program including activity, medication, rest, exercise, and diet to make sure you get the maximum improvement.

If you have osteoporosis, the earlier you care for it, the better the results of treatment will be. This treatment can be started by you, today, in your own home, along with the help of your physician.

If you find that you have osteoporosis, don't panic! A positive attitude is one of the most important weapons you can have to improve your outcome. Positive thinking is free and has no side effects. An important part of a patient's treatment depends on the individual's outlook.

Case Study

We recently had as a patient a preretirement woman who suffered fractures in her spine that resulted in constant pain in the middle and lower back. She gradually became severely limited in standing and walking, and she was forced to give up her job as a cashier where she was on her feet all day. The patient was determined to manage her illness and began a prescribed program of exercise, rest, and medications. Over a period of a few months, the patient was able to walk with little or no pain. She was able to return to work. Through determination and hard work, she was able to regain her income and most likely avoided becoming disabled with many more medical problems.

You Are the Key in Treatment

In our clinic, we encourage patients to approach this problem of osteoporosis in an orderly way. The confusing combination of pain, stiffness, and limitation of movement can now be correctly diagnosed. Patients can begin treatment knowing which treatments of exercise, rest, and medications have the best chance for success.

You can and must become an expert in your own specific problem with osteoporosis and begin the best possible treatments immediately. You need accurate information about the causes, the available treatment, and what the future is expected to be for you.

This book will give you the information you need to take an active part in your own treatment—managing your osteoporosis. This will allow you to manage your osteoporosis the same as you manage other areas of your life and to live an active life without fear of fractures.

=============== **SUMMARY** ===============

1. Osteoporosis is the thinning of bones—a decrease in the density of the bones.
2. Osteoporosis begins silently. By age 65, as many as 80 percent of women may have osteoporosis, and 25 percent may have fractures. Up to 20 percent of women in their 40s may have osteoporosis.
3. Over 1,500,000 fractures happen in the United States each year due to osteoporosis with a cost of $10 billion.
4. Twenty percent of patients with fractures of the hip from osteoporosis may not walk after one year, and 20 percent may die within one year.
5. Prevention and treatments for many causes of osteoporosis are now available. There is effective treatment that can increase the bone density and lower the chance of future fractures.
6. We have a choice. We can continue to treat only fractures in hips, spines, and other bones and watch the increase in costs of personal health care. Or, we can use prevention and treatment to lower the risk of future fractures, resulting in great savings in cost and suffering.

CHAPTER TWO

The Risk Factors: Are You a Candidate for Osteoporosis?

Although osteoporosis can have severe consequences, prevention and treatment can begin if detected early. Some people are at much higher risk for osteoporosis and fracture than others. This higher risk may result in a hip fracture, fracture of the spine, or wrist fracture much earlier than the usual age of 50 or more. Risk factors for osteoporosis can be easily detected. The more risk factors you have, the greater your chances of getting osteoporosis. Once identified, these risk factors can be reduced and you can begin to lessen your chances of having osteoporosis and fractures in the future. It is never too early to start prevention for osteoporosis since this process may begin well before age 40.

If you have more than one or two risk factors, your chances of future osteoporosis are too significant to ignore. In fact, the more risk factors you have, the higher the chance of future fractures and the greater need for earlier action on your part.

Let's review these risk factors. Chapters Five and Six will explain how you can manage these factors to prevent and treat osteoporosis.

Risk Factors

1. Lack of regular exercise program
2. In women, menopause, especially early menopause
3. Age 40 or older
4. Female
5. White
6. Cigarette smoking
7. Family members who have osteoporosis
8. Underweight for your height
9. Heavy alcohol use
10. Certain medications: Cortisone-like drugs, Aluminum-containing antacids
11. Certain medical problems, such as:
    Rheumatoid arthritis
    Emphysema, chronic bronchitis
    Hyperthyroidism
    Some types of stomach surgery
    Diabetes mellitus
12. Low calcium in diet
13. Injuries and falls

Lack of Regular Exercise Program

Regular exercise does help to delay or even reverse the process of osteoporosis. This has been shown to be true in animal experiments where changes in the amount of strain on bones resulted in changes in the structure of bones. It is possible that exercise stimulates the cells in bones which make new bone so that even more bone is formed.

On the other hand, lack of exercise is well established as an important risk factor and cause of osteoporosis. It has been known for many years that patients who must have prolonged inactivity or bedrest for other reasons often develop osteoporosis. The exact reason is not known. However, it seems that activity, especially weight-bearing activity, in some way stimulates bone cells to be more active and to produce stronger bone. Without activity, bones may become less dense and weaker. Some researchers have found that after prolonged bedrest it may take months for bone to become normal again even if no other problems are present.

More recently, extensive studies performed on astronauts have shown there is a major problem in longer space flights due to the inactivity and weightlessness which cause loss of bone density. This is in healthy astronauts! Researchers are now trying to find ways to deal with this problem.

Physically active people have denser bones compared to inactive people of the same age. Studies in animals show changes in the amount of strain on bones result in changes in the structure of bones. Conclusions from recent research show that one of the strongest natural stimulations for bone formation is weight-bearing activities such as walking or running.

After age 30 to 40, many people become less physically active. This is often a result of their more sedentary work and a general decline in physical conditioning that is common in these years. In people over age 50, it is even more common to see decreases in physical activity. The gradual decrease in exercise, especially weight-bearing exercise over a period of years, results in less stimulation for bone formation. This occurs in years when other risk factors may also be at work to weaken bone.

In older people, the tendency to have less and less exercise is a greater problem. If other medical problems or a fracture cause even less activity, it is easy to see how osteoporosis may worsen rapidly.

Lack of exercise is a major risk factor, but it is also easy to correct with a simple walking program. Most of the patients we see with fractures from osteoporosis were not aware that activity such as walking would improve bone strength. Almost every patient is able to help by beginning a simple weight-bearing exercise program under his or her physician's direction.

Exercises to build other muscles that give support to the body are also important. However, the specific relationship to the risk of osteoporosis is not known. It seems reasonable to assume that stronger muscles would give more support to the bones. Exercises for the back and other muscles are discussed in Chapter Seven.

A word of caution: It is possible to get too much exercise. It has been found that some women (mainly young athletes) who exercise very strenuously for a prolonged period may develop fractures. This type of exercise results in hormonal changes that cause a change or stoppage of the menstrual periods. As you will learn in the next section, such a change may result in osteoporosis as well. This can lead to fractures in the feet and legs of runners. Adjusting training or adding medication can usually control this problem. Overall this problem is uncommon.

You can get a good indication of how much weight-bearing exercise you perform regularly by completing the exercise chart below for one week (Table 2). The amount of exercise needed to prevent osteoporosis is not known. In our clinic, we suggest 30 to 40 minutes of weight-bearing exercise several times a week. This includes walking, bicycle riding, running, jumping rope, or climbing stairs. For those patients who are unable to get out-of-doors on weekdays, an exercise bicycle may be a wise investment for future good health.

If you have been physically inactive for a long time, do not begin with 30 minutes of strenuous exercise. Moderation is the key in starting any new conditioning program. A reasonable

TABLE 2
Daily Exercise Chart

	A.M.							P.M.									
	6	7	8	9	10	11	12	1	2	3	4	5	6	7	8	9	10
Monday																	
Tuesday																	
Wednesday																	
Thursday																	
Friday																	
Saturday																	
Sunday																	

Check off the times of day you perform weight-bearing exercises, including walking, stair-climbing, jumping rope, bicycle riding, running, or other exercise to total 30 to 40 minutes several times each week. Try to include times for exercise in your daily routine such as walking to the store, taking the stairs, parking at the *back* of the parking lot.

exercise routine may include a 10-minute walk every other day for a week or two. As your body adjusts to the new exercise routine, add 5 more minutes to this walk. Try this for another week or two. Allow yourself at least 2 months to build up to the goal of 30 to 40 minutes of weight-bearing exercise. Remember, it is better to begin slowly at a reasonable pace than to have to stop completely due to injury.

Many people say they do not have time to exercise due to their daily responsibilities. But if the ultimate reward is avoiding osteoporosis, then these people must view exercise as a part of the prescription for their good health. Other benefits of a regular exercise program include strengthening and toning muscles. When the spine is more stable, back pain is less likely to occur. Exercise can also lower your blood pressure and resting heart rate while strengthening your overall cardiovascular system. The benefits of a regular exercise program including weight-bearing exercise such as walking, climbing stairs, or jumping rope, are too important to your overall health to be ignored.

Make time in your schedule to perform weight-bearing exercises just as you make time to eat, dress, or read the newspaper. (See Table 2.) Read Chapter Seven for a description of some of these exercises.

Menopause in Women

There is a much higher risk of osteoporosis after menopause in women. The risk increases if you happen to be affected by early natural menopause in which the menstrual periods stop at an earlier age than the average age of 45 to 55, or if you have had both ovaries removed by surgery.

Ovaries are the organs that produce one of the female hormones, estrogen. The female hormone system, especially estrogen, is important in bone formation. At menopause, the ovaries produce less estrogen so the amount of estrogen in the body decreases. Although the process is not very well understood, lower estrogen levels in some way cause less bone formation, increase the amount of bone lost, with the result that the bones gradually become thinner.

If menopause happens earlier in life, it may allow osteo-porosis to begin earlier. Why some women reach menopause earlier than others is not known. It is known, however, that such women are at greater risk of developing osteoporosis. If the ovaries are removed surgically, the source of estrogen is also re-moved. One common operation in which the ovaries are some-times removed is a hysterectomy (removal of the uterus). The reasons for ovary removal are varied; when possible, however, most surgeons try to leave one ovary in place to allow estrogen hormone production to continue as long as possible. In that situation, the decrease in estrogen level would probably be be-tween ages 45 to 55.

The problem crucial to women and osteoporosis is that once the lower levels of estrogen cause osteoporosis and bone is lost, the body is quite limited in its ability to actually re-place the lost bone. Therefore, this risk factor, which is the ma-jor factor in osteoporosis in most women, must be detected early so that any possible treatment might be started as soon after menopause as possible. The recommended treatment is discussed in Chapter Six.

Age and Sex

After we reach maturity, there is a gradual decrease in the total amount of bone formed compared to the amount re-moved. Sometime after age 30 to 40 there is a gradual loss of bone density. This happens more rapidly in women than in men. At first, the change in bone formation and removal is very gradual and is not detectable. In fact, we are not able to detect it even with our most sensitive tests until there is loss of a fairly large amount of bone. By age 60, many women may have lost 20 percent or more of the amount of bone which was present at age 30. In men, the loss of bone is much slower.

Until there is a better way to tell when this very gradual change in bone density happens, we can only predict a higher risk of this process happening in people over age 35 to 40, espe-cially in women. Although we can't change age or sex, there are other risk factors that can be adequately controlled to keep this particular risk to a minimum.

Race

Osteoporosis is more common in people of the Caucasian race who have fair complexions. African-Americans have more dense bones and a less rapid loss of bone once this process begins. The reason for this protective effect is not known. In some way, African-Americans seem to have a genetic "program" for more dense bones.

In fact, Caucasian women have about twice as many hip fractures as African-American women. The rate of bone loss and risk of osteoporosis are therefore highest in Caucasian women and lowest in African-American men. Persons of Asian origin may have an intermediate risk of getting the disease.

Cigarette Smoking

Smoking cigarettes doubles your risk of osteoporosis. Researchers have found that osteoporosis happens earlier and continues more rapidly in smokers than in nonsmokers. The reason for this is not known. Substances in cigarettes cause a number of chemical and hormonal changes in the body that may result in earlier and more severe osteoporosis. In addition, some smokers tend to be underweight which increases the risk of osteoporosis.

The good news about cigarette smoking as a risk factor is that you can do something to eliminate the problem. There are many painless methods to enable smokers to give up the habit entirely. Prescription patches are available that can help ease the withdrawal symptoms common to smokers.

If you are a smoker, you are at high risk for osteoporosis. As a smoker, you are also at risk for heart disease, lung cancer, emphysema, hardening of the arteries, and other diseases. Work with your physician to quit the habit. Recruit a support system of family and friends to help you get through the first few days, then enjoy improved health as cigarettes no longer are a part of your daily habit.

Genetics: Family History of Osteoporosis

The adage "like mother, like daughter" runs quite true with osteoporosis. There seems to be a higher risk of osteoporosis if you have other natural family members who are affected by this disease. The reasons are not known, but it is likely that this is due to the inherited genetic "program" that somehow makes a person more susceptible. If you have a family member who has suffered from "soft bones," frequent fractures, loss of height, and stooped posture, you should be aware that you are at higher than average risk. And if you have other risk factors, you should take proper precautions to prevent osteoporosis.

Thin or Heavy

Women who are underweight for their height often develop osteoporosis more rapidly. Women who are overweight have less chance of osteoporosis. It is possible that more fat tissue results in more production of the female estrogen hormones. This higher level of estrogens could slow the process of osteoporosis. Of course, being overweight increases the risk of other medical problems. We do not recommend weight gain to prevent osteoporosis unless you are underweight. (See Table 3 on pp. 29–30.)

Heavy Alcohol Use

Over the past few years, it has been recognized that people who drink alcohol in heavy amounts have a higher risk of osteoporosis. The amount of alcohol intake to cause this problem is not known. It seems to occur mainly with heavy use. It is not thought that smaller amounts of alcohol increase the risk osteoporosis. For example, it seems likely that moderate amounts of alcohol (such as 1 ounce of 80 proof distilled liquor, a 12 oz. beer, or less than half a bottle of wine a day) do not greatly increase the risk. Heavier intake of alcohol for a number of years does increase the risk.

Heavy drinkers may have osteoporosis at a much younger age than usual. In fact, the disease can be seen in people as young as ages 30 to 40. It may be seen in men as well as women even though osteoporosis is usually much more common in women. This risk factor may easily be overlooked as a cause of osteoporosis and pain.

TABLE 3
Metropolitan Height and Weight Tables
MEN

| Height | | Small | Medium | Large |
Feet	Inches	Frame	Frame	Frame
5	2	128–134	131–141	138–150
5	3	130–136	133–143	140–153
5	4	132–138	135–145	142–156
5	5	134–140	137–148	144–160
5	6	136–142	139–151	146–164
5	7	138–145	142–154	149–168
5	8	140–148	145–157	152–172
5	9	142–151	148–160	155–176
5	10	144–154	151–163	158–180
5	11	146–157	154–166	161–184
6	0	149–160	157–170	164–188
6	1	152–164	160–174	168–192
6	2	155–168	164–178	172–197
6	3	158–172	167–182	176–202
6	4	162–176	171-187	181–207

Weights at Ages 25–59 Based on Lowest Mortality. Weight in Pounds According to Frame (in indoor clothing weighing 5 lbs., shoes with 1″ heels).

Source of basic data: *1979 Build Study*, Society of Actuaries and Association of Life Insurance Medical Directors of America, 1980. Reprinted with permission from Metropolitan Life Insurance Company, New York, New York.

Certain Medications

Certain medications taken for other reasons may increase your risk of osteoporosis. One of the most common is the group of cortisone-like drugs (Table 4). These medicines increase the chance of osteoporosis if taken regularly, especially if taken over a long period of time. The risk increases with higher doses and longer time of treatment. If these medicines are taken for a short period of time (such as days or a few weeks), then there need be no great concern about osteoporosis.

These medicines are often used in short courses for problems such as allergic reactions, asthma, bursitis, and other

TABLE 3 (continued)
WOMEN

Height Feet	Inches	Small Frame	Medium Frame	Large Frame
4	10	102–111	109–121	118–131
4	11	103–113	111–123	120–134
5	0	104–115	113–126	122–137
5	1	106–118	115–129	125–140
5	2	108–121	118–132	128–143
5	3	111–124	121–135	131–147
5	4	114–127	124–138	134–151
5	5	117–130	127–141	137–155
5	6	120–133	130–144	140–159
5	7	123–136	133–147	143–163
5	8	126–139	136–150	146–167
5	9	129–142	139–153	149–170
5	10	132–145	142–156	152–173
5	11	135–148	145–159	155–176
6	0	138–151	148–162	158–179

Weights at Ages 25–59 Based on Lowest Mortality. Weight in Pounds According to Frame (in indoor clothing weighing 3 lbs., shoes with 1" heels).

Source of basic data: 1979 Build Study, Society of Actuaries and Association of Life Insurance Medical Directors of America, 1980. Reprinted with permission from Metropolitan Life Insurance Company, New York, New York.

problems that are not long-lasting. These cortisone-like medicines may also be needed for more long-lasting problems. Higher doses may be needed to control some diseases such as severe lung disease. If these higher doses are used over a long time (such as months or years), then the risk of osteoporosis increases. Such medications can lower the absorption of calcium from the intestine. As a result, lower amounts of calcium are available to the body. Then more bone may be removed by the body to make more calcium available. With the use of cortisone-like drugs, the activity of cells that produce bone is decreased. Overall, these medications seem to increase bone loss and decrease bone formation.

TABLE 4
Common Cortisone-Like Drugs

Generic Name	Brand Name
Betamethasone	Celestone
Dexamethasone	Decadron
Methylprednisolone	Medrol
Prednisolone	Delta-Cortef
Prednisone	Deltasone
	Orasone
Triamcinolone	Aristocort

Diseases That May Be Treated with One of These Drugs

Asthma	Some skin diseases
Acute bronchitis	Allergic reactions
Chronic bronchitis	Some eye diseases
Rheumatoid arthritis	Ulcerative colitis
Systemic lupus erythematosus	Some blood diseases
Arthritis of other types	Some cases of leukemia

Another way in which cortisone-like medicines are used is by local injection. This treatment may be used in bursitis, tendinitis, and some forms of arthritis. These injections do not raise the risk of osteoporosis. In fact, the great advantage of the local injection is that relief of pain is usually fast and without significant side effects. Your physician may guide you in your situation.

Certain Medical Problems

Rheumatoid Arthritis

Rheumatoid arthritis is one of the most common kinds of arthritis in young women. Overall, it affects up to 1 to 2 percent of the population and can be quite severe. Rheumatoid arthritis causes pain and swelling in the joints, often involving the hands, wrists, elbows, shoulders, knees, ankles, and feet. Stiffness in the joints, especially in the morning, and fatigue may be severe. Fever and weight loss may occur. Many daily activities such as walking and the use of the hands are difficult.

A person with rheumatoid arthritis has a higher risk of developing osteoporosis. Arthritis pain makes activity and regular exercise harder, especially walking and other weight-bearing exercise. This lack of regular exercise increases the risk of osteoporosis. Some patients with rheumatoid arthritis are treated with cortisone-like drugs which also increase the risk of osteoporosis. There are probably some other unknown causes as a result of the disease itself that contribute to osteoporosis in rheumatoid arthritis. Unfortunately, osteoporosis does affect a large portion of patients with rheumatoid arthritis. This may cause interference with treatment of the arthritis if fractures occur. The arthritis may make surgery involving bones and joints more complicated. The disease is so common in rheumatoid patients that these individuals must take extra care in prevention and treatment of osteoporosis.

Emphysema, Chronic Bronchitis

Many patients with lung disease, especially emphysema and chronic bronchitis related to cigarette smoking, have osteoporosis. In emphysema, there is a loss of lung tissue which results in shortness of breath and limitation of physical activities. This disease may be slowly progressive over many years. In chronic bronchitis, there is inflammation of the bronchial tubes that results in increased secretions and cough. Chronic bronchitis also causes shortness of breath that may restrict physical activity. The most common cause of these diseases is cigarette smoking. As in rheumatoid arthritis, there are probably a number of other factors that are important. Cigarettes alone increase the risk, as we have discussed. Smokers who are underweight are at an increased risk as well. The level of oxygen in the blood is often decreased in these patients because of the lung disease. This lower level of oxygen may affect the way the body builds and removes bone. As a result of these factors, a person is generally at a much higher risk for osteoporosis if emphysema and chronic bronchitis are present. Osteoporosis is so common in this situation that these patients should also take extra care to control other risk factors and take special care for the prevention and treatment of the disease.

Diabetes Mellitus

Some researchers have found that patients who are "diabetic" have a higher chance of developing osteoporosis. The millions of Americans who have diabetes mellitus are at a higher risk for osteoporosis.

Hyperthyroidism

This is a condition of overactivity of the thyroid gland. Too much thyroid hormone is produced by the thyroid. The most common early symptoms are nervousness, weight loss, and rapid heart rate. Another result of this thyroid overactivity is osteoporosis. Hyperthyroidism can be diagnosed and treated by your physician.

Stomach (Gastric) Surgery

Peptic ulcer disease and other conditions may require surgery involving removal of a portion of the stomach. In some cases, a higher chance of developing osteoporosis has been found. If you have had stomach surgery, then follow your physician's advice for specific ways to adjust your diet or food supplements to minimize your risk.

Uncommon Medical Problems

Uncommon medical problems may also cause osteoporosis. Hyperparathyroidism is overactivity of the parathyroid glands located in the neck. These glands produce parathyroid hormone that is important in the control of bone removal in the body. Excessive levels of this hormone result in rapid bone loss. This condition can be diagnosed and treated by a physician.

There are other uncommon or rare medical problems that cause or aggravate osteoporosis. These are best found by a physician and require treatment to remove the higher risk.

Low Calcium in the Diet

If your diet has been consistently low in calcium over the years, especially during the growth years, there is a higher risk of osteoporosis. Adolescents with a diet low in calcium for a number of years have less bone formed. Then, when the rate of bone loss becomes greater than the rate of bone formation, osteoporosis occurs more quickly. (See Table 5 for the recommended daily allowance of calcium for infants through adults.)

Although low calcium in the body contributes to the development of osteoporosis, you cannot treat osteoporosis with only calcium supplementation. Refer to Chapter Five on treatment of osteoporosis to see the designated combination of vitamins, minerals, prescription drugs, and exercise for your specific stage of osteoporosis.

Some persons do not tolerate the lactose in milk and some milk products. Because of this, they avoid milk products and dairy foods. As a result, calcium intake may be low for years. This problem can be managed in several ways as discussed in Chapter Four.

Weight-control diets may contain low amounts of calcium. Careful attention to content of calcium and other nutrients while dieting can eliminate this risk factor. This is discussed in Chapter Four. Older patients above 65 years of age need a higher dose of calcium because the intestine absorbs calcium less efficiently.

TABLE 5
Recommended Daily Dietary
Allowance for Calcium

Age		Allowance
Infant:	0–6 months	360 mg
	6–12 months	540 mg
Children:	1–3 years	800 mg
	4–6 years	800 mg
	7–10 years	800 mg
Teenagers:	11–18 years	1200 mg
Pregnant teens:	11–18 years	1600 mg
Pregnant women:	19 +	1200 mg
Lactating women:	19 +	1200 mg
Adults:	19 +	1000 mg

Injuries and Falls

It makes sense that if bones become weak then less injury is required to cause a fracture. Enough bone is lost in Stage 3 and Stage 4 osteoporosis so that injuries and falls result in fractures of bones. Prevention of falls and injuries in persons of high risk or with known osteoporosis would be very helpful.

Physical problems in such persons range from unsteadiness, weakness in muscles, dizziness, heart problems, to medications that can cause unsteadiness.

Other problems that cause falls and injuries are often difficult to identify and at times are simply a result of being unlucky. Tripping over objects such as furniture, telephone cords, and rugs are problems at home that might be avoided if considered carefully. Good lighting, especially at night, in an elderly person's home may also result in less frequent falls and limit this risk factor.

This risk factor is important for those persons who have osteoporosis and are at high risk for fracture (Stages 3 and 4). Remember, less injury is needed to cause a fracture in these

TABLE 6
Safe Living

By taking control over your home and work environment, you can avoid unexpected falls or injuries.

Let the following checklist serve as a reminder to take care of unsafe situations before a fall leads to a fracture or broken bone.

Home Entrance

- Sidewalk or stones level
- Toys and lawn equipment put away
- Water hoses coiled or placed next to house
- Doormats flat on ground level with no turned up edges
- Step-up into home at reasonable level and easy to see
- Porch and outside lighting adequate

Living Room

- All electrical cords placed next to wall or behind furniture
- Ample walk-through space without blockage of furniture

(continued)

TABLE 6 *(continued)*

- Rugs flat on floor and anchored down or with nonskid mats under them
- Tile level
- Avoid all waxes or floor shines that may cause slippery floors

Bedroom

- Bedspread or dust ruffle at least 1" off floor to avoid tripping
- Bed pulled away from wall for easy access when changing linens
- Electrical cords placed behind furniture
- Shoes organized in shoebag hanging in closet
- All accessories at easy-to-reach level and organized on shelves
- Well-lit

Bathroom

- Flat, nonskid rug on floor to avoid slipping
- Nonskid bathmat in tub or shower
- Easy-to-reach shelf in tub or shower for bath products and soaps
- Liquid soaps to avoid slipping on bars
- Well-lit
- Nightlight
- Medicines used frequently on lowest shelf in cabinet
- Grab bars in shower and by toilet

Kitchen

- Nonskid mat by sink
- Smooth floor to avoid tripping
- Avoid floor wax and shine products
- Place items rarely used on top shelves
- Store pots and pans at easy reach level
- Stack plastic and glass items on lower shelves
- Have equipment used daily such as plates, bowls, glasses, and pans stored at waist to eye level to avoid straining
- Make sure kitchen table and chairs are well-balanced

The three important factors to remember when practicing safe living are:

1. Go slow—falls may occur when you hurry
2. Think before you move—often carelessness adds to your risk of injury
3. Take charge of your environment—make certain you have followed the suggested safety guidelines.

stages. Minor falls that would have gone unnoticed years earlier may result in a fracture of a wrist, hip, spine, or other bone. Since some of these falls and injuries may be preventable, it is especially useful to spend some time making the living situation as safe as possible. Look at Table 6 and check those areas that need inspection in your home.

A thorough knowledge of risk factors is necessary for prevention of osteoporosis. The next chapter discusses the signs and symptoms of osteoporosis as it develops and progresses.

SUMMARY

1. Osteoporosis is not random—some persons are at much higher risk for osteoporosis and fractures.
2. Risk factors include:
   Lack of regular exercise program
   Menopause in women, especially early menopause
   Age 40 or over
   Female
   White
   Cigarette smoking
   Family members who have osteoporosis
   Underweight for your height
   Heavy alcohol use
   Certain medications
   Certain medical problems
   Low calcium in diet
   Injuries and falls
3. Knowledge of risk factors allows prevention and treatment.
4. If you have more than 1 or 2 risk factors, you should consider further specific prevention.
5. The earlier prevention is started, the more effective it can be. Prevention of osteoporosis can begin in children.

CHAPTER THREE

The Four Stages: Diagnosis and Detection

The best treatment for osteoporosis is prevention. After osteoporosis is present, it will progress through several stages. Treatment at each stage may delay or stop more severe osteoporosis and fractures. Let's discuss the signs and symptoms of osteoporosis—and how the diagnosis is made. You will be able to tell into which stage your situation best fits. In Chapters Four and Five, you will see how you can begin to prevent and manage each stage of osteoporosis.

Stage 1:
Before Osteoporosis Is Detectable

Stage 1 usually begins some time after reaching young adult age, often beginning between age 30 and 40. There are no feelings or signs for you to tell that the process is beginning. In fact, no X-ray or other readily available test can detect this stage effectively. If you have more than one or two of the risk factors then it is reasonable to begin prevention measures as outlined in Chapter Four.

How can you tell if this gradual process has begun? How can you tell if the process that will eventually lead to osteoporosis has started in your body? It is not possible to tell in an individual just when this process starts. But if you wait until diagnosis is possible to begin specific measures for prevention, you will lose many valuable years. Since we can tell which persons are at a higher risk for osteoporosis, these persons should act as if Stage 1 osteoporosis has begun. This will allow you to take reasonable steps to allow removal of risk factors and hopefully delay or prevent osteoporosis. It is true that some persons with risk factors may not develop osteoporosis. However, a large number of those with several risk factors will have osteoporosis. Until more discoveries about the causes of osteoporosis are made, it is safest to start specific preventive measures if you have more than two risk factors. Remember the serious and potentially devastating results of osteoporosis when untreated over many years.

Let's consider an example of a person who may be in Stage 1 osteoporosis. We recently saw a 41-year-old woman who was concerned about her chances of osteoporosis. She had read that osteoporosis may run in families. Her mother and grandmother both had early menopause (around age 44) and suffered fractures in their early 50s. Her grandmother had become stooped in posture and broke her hip in a fall. Her grandmother was now living in a nursing home.

This woman also had avoided dairy products since a teenager as part of a continuing low-calorie diet. She had smoked cigarettes for about 10 years.

Let's look at the risk factors present. This woman was over 40, smoked cigarettes, had a strong family history of osteoporosis, and probably has had a low-calcium intake for years. She certainly would be at a higher risk for osteoporosis in the future. She is at an excellent point to begin specific preventive measures since she is in Stage 1 osteoporosis. She needs to stop cigarette smoking, begin a weight-bearing exercise program, increase calcium in the diet as suggested in Chapter Four, and maintain a normal body weight for her bone structure. (See Table 3, p. 30.) These preventive measures are simple and inexpensive. They will also add benefits to her overall health. Steps taken now could make a big difference years from now in preventing fractures. It is an investment that could pay great dividends in the future.

Stage 2:
Osteoporosis Becomes Detectable

Between ages 35 and 55, depending on the number of risk factors present, osteoporosis will become detectable. There are still no feelings and no outward signs since it is early in the course of the disease. But there are several other ways to detect osteoporosis at this point.

If you have an X-ray taken for other reasons, ask your physician to see if there is evidence of osteoporosis present in the bones. Because X-rays are taken for many reasons, these X-rays may not always help. But if osteoporosis does happen to be detectable, it would be very important to know. Treatment, as outlined in Chapter Six, can begin. One problem with using regular X-rays is that up to 30 percent of bone density must be lost before it becomes very detectable.

In the past few years, researchers have made available to most physicians and hospitals several newer and much more accurate tests to detect osteoporosis. These tests measure the density of the bones directly. The test can accurately tell how much, if any, osteoporosis is present and can help give an estimate of the risk of fractures. These tests can detect osteoporosis much earlier than standard X-rays, often years before fractures occur.

Usually the bone density of the hip, spine, or lower arm near the wrist is measured. These areas are thought to represent the other bones of the body without going to the expense of measuring each bone.

There are several types of bone density tests available. Some tests involve additional radiation exposure, and some tests are not as accurate as others. The newest tests (called dual energy X-ray) are easy to take and are not painful. They have almost no extra radiation exposure and are considered by many to be the best test available. The information obtained is very helpful to guide treatment. However, no test can perfectly predict whether a fracture will happen.

Some practitioners have suggested that all women over 40 years old should have a bone density test to detect osteoporosis. This would be very expensive since there are over 60 million women over 40 in the United States.

When should you consider having a bone density test? Here are some practical suggestions to gain the most information possible about osteoporosis with the least expense, risk, and trouble.

1. If osteoporosis is already definitely established by a fracture on X-ray (Stage 3 or 4), the value of the test is that it will tell the severity of osteoporosis and help guide treatment. This is important since treatments are available that work. The test may be repeated in 1 or 2 years to measure the amount of improvement.

2. If you have several risk factors for osteoporosis and plan to repeat the test in 1 or 2 years for comparison, it is reasonable to have a bone density test. If it does not show the presence of osteoporosis, then prevention measures can be continued.

3. The results of the test might help to decide a different treatment for you. For example, a patient or physician may wish to avoid higher calcium in the diet, estrogen treatment, or other medications. In this situation, a test result that showed no osteoporosis might allow delay in beginning some treatments. If severe osteoporosis is present, the bone density test may allow treatment to begin earlier, when it will be most useful to prevent fractures.

4. Persons with many risk factors might wish to have all the information possible for peace of mind.

5. Some medical problems and some medications, such as cortisone medications can cause osteoporosis. It may be helpful to measure bone density when these are first started to allow early treatment if osteoporosis develops.

Let's now consider an example of a person in Stage 2 osteoporosis. A woman was recently seen in our clinic who was 49 years old, white, had smoked cigarettes for 15 years, and has had rheumatoid arthritis for 10 years. The arthritis was quite severe at times and interfered with her work as a hairdresser. She had taken prednisone (a cortisone-like drug) for months at a time over the 10 years so that she could have relief from the arthritis and continue to work.

This woman came to her physician because the pain of arthritis had become severe. She became more concerned about future osteoporosis when she learned about the risk factors. She has the risk factors of being over 40, female, white, smoking cigarettes, having rheumatoid arthritis, and treatment with a cortisone-like drug. If this woman suffered a fracture over the next few years, it would not be surprising! She had a bone density test performed and was found to have significant osteoporosis although she had no visible symptoms. She has osteoporosis, Stage 2, and has begun a program of treatment. Hopefully her actions now will prevent fractures and suffering years from now. How do we know that this woman will have a fracture if she is not treated? We do not know that fact, but it does make sense that if we are ever to prevent the loss of bone density that results in osteoporosis, it would be best to start early before fractures happen. It is hoped that researchers will be able to tell in the future which people with risk factors will actually develop osteoporosis.

Stage 3:
Osteoporosis Results in Fractures

In Stage 3 osteoporosis, a fracture has happened. This may be from a minor fall or strain. The first realization of osteoporosis may come with a fracture. As you can see, this is not early in the course of osteoporosis. The fracture heals and the pain usually goes away completely. It is important that the osteoporosis that increased the opportunity for the fracture be detected. If the osteoporosis is not treated, more fractures are likely and progression to Stage 4 may happen.

This may be the most common stage in which osteoporosis is recognized. A fracture happens with or without a serious injury or fall. Especially if the injury seems minor, it is a good idea to specifically look for evidence of osteoporosis on an X-ray. This can sometimes be done using the X-rays taken for the fracture.

If osteoporosis is diagnosed after a fracture, then it would represent Stage 3 osteoporosis. It is likely that it has been present for years. But since it caused no signs or symptoms, it was not detected. Sometimes there may be more than one fracture before osteoporosis is detected.

We recently saw a woman, aged 50, who had suffered a broken ankle in a fall at work. Her physician thought the fracture was more serious than one might usually see for that injury. It turned out that this woman had osteoporosis which probably contributed to the severity of the fracture. She began treatment of Stage 3 osteoporosis, hopefully to prevent future fractures.

Another woman was seen who was 60 at the time. She suffered a fracture of the shoulder (humerus) when she was involved in an automobile accident. Then, the diagnosis of osteoporosis was made when an X-ray was taken because of the shoulder injury. A bone density test to measure the severity of osteoporosis was done. If the bone density is low, it seems reasonable to suspect that the slightest injury could cause a fracture.

You have probably heard of a person, especially an older person, who had a fracture after an apparent minor injury. Bone density tests are important so you can tell if osteoporosis is present.

Stage 4:
Osteoporosis with Chronic Pain
and Deformity

As more fractures happen, the pain may become constant. Fractures will heal, but deformities can begin. Most common are deformities of the back with a stooped appearance (see Figure 6, p. 8).

Loss of ability to walk from fracture of a hip can happen in either Stage 3 or 4. Research has found in elderly people, up to 50 percent who fracture a hip aren't able to walk as they could before, and up to 20 percent may die the first year.

Stage 4 usually happens after age 55. The familiar stooped appearance can happen in women and men. The stooped appearance may cause no pain, but often the fractures cause pain and limitation of activity.

Let's look at a few examples of Stage 4 osteoporosis. We saw a man who was 63 years old and who had a serious illness that required high doses of cortisone-like drugs. This allowed the man to recover from his medical problem. The man also smoked cigarettes for many years, was thin and underweight, and had quite limited activity for a few years due to his other medical problems. One year earlier, the man developed severe back pain that was also felt in his right and left side. He had great trouble standing and walking because of the severe pain. He was awakened at night by the back pain that hurt even when taking a deep breath. The pain gradually improved and went away after a few months.

After he became active again, the man developed severe lower back pain. He was again unable to walk. After 6 months of pain, he was found to have a number of fractures in the spine that had caused him to become stooped in appearance. He uses a walker when outside of his home. It is hoped that as he becomes stronger, he will be less limited. He continues treatment to try to prevent future fractures.

We saw a 65-year-old woman who had several fractures in the spine from osteoporosis. She was in constant pain for over a year and lost 2 inches in height. She began treatment for osteoporosis and, after two years, she returned to her job which required standing for more than six hours each day. She has become virtually pain-free.

Unfortunately, success stories are only one side. A most unfortunate outcome happened in one woman with severe osteoporosis. She had a large number of risk factors for many years and developed fractures in the spine with severe, constant pain. She was unable to walk or care for herself and became discouraged and depressed because progress seemed so slow. Her husband developed other serious medical problems as well. This couple took their own lives in a moment of despair.

The signs and symptoms of osteoporosis are late in appearance. It is not recommended or useful to wait until there are symptoms of osteoporosis. If you have risk factors, you should be aware of the need for early prevention, detection, and treatment. Bone density testing can guide treatment.

It is hoped that future research will allow better treatment of severe and advanced cases of osteoporosis. Until then, we should concentrate on prevention and treatment as early as possible. It is never too early to begin prevention and never too late to treat osteoporosis.

Chapters Four and Five will show you how to manage osteoporosis with guidelines for prevention and treatment.

═══════════   SUMMARY   ═══════════

1. Stage 1 and Stage 2 have no symptoms. Stage 2 is detectable by bone density tests before fractures happen.
2. Stage 3 symptoms and signs are from fractures of bones.
3. Stage 4 symptoms and signs result from more fractures with pain and deformities.
4. Signs and symptoms of osteoporosis are late in appearance and allow diagnosis only after it is advanced. Knowledge of risk factors allows early prevention, detection, and treatment.
5. Bone density tests can be used to measure the severity of osteoporosis and to guide treatment.

CHAPTER FOUR

A Prevention Plan for Osteoporosis

Osteoporosis has no known cure. But prevention measures may reduce or even halt the bone loss. The earlier you begin to manage your lifestyle for prevention of osteoporosis, the more effective the results will be. Action taken at an early stage of the disease may produce better results than the same action taken later in the course of osteoporosis.

The prevention measures suggested in this book do not require a drastic change in lifestyle. In fact, most of our patients are able to incorporate a daily program of weight-bearing exercise, vitamins, and a calcium-rich diet into their schedules without many complaints. Most patients report that even though the measures are suggested to help prevent osteoporosis, their overall well-being is improved as diet and activity changes are made.

You can decide to take an active part in starting this management when it will be the most useful to produce the greatest benefits. The best rule of thumb is to begin now.

Stage 1:
Before Osteoporosis Is Detectable

Stage 1 osteoporosis may begin sometime after a person has reached maturity, which usually happens around age 20 or 30. The time of rapid growth and formation of bones from childhood and adolescence is decreasing. The rate of bone formation begins to slowly decrease. The rate of bone removal may stay the same or slightly increase. As a result of these changes, very gradually the total amount of bone formed becomes slightly less compared to the total amount of bone removed. Over a period of years, this may result in a gradual decrease in the amount of bone density, which results in osteoporosis.

It is not known exactly what makes this process happen faster in one person than in another. But we do know that some people seem to be at more risk for this problem than others. After many years, the bones eventually become weak enough so that fractures happen. Usually this is the time when we first suspect osteoporosis.

It would be best if we could tell which people have begun this process of less bone formation compared to more bone removal. Then, ideally we would somehow correct the process at that point while the bones are strong. The problem is that not enough is known at this time to allow such treatment. Hopefully, researchers will soon have more answers.

Since it is possible to tell which people are probably at higher risk for osteoporosis, it seems reasonable to try to change some of the risk factors which we do know about. By removing as many risk factors as possible, the chance of later development of osteoporosis may be decreased. This would allow prevention of osteoporosis rather than waiting for fractures to begin treatment. It is apparent that if people continue to wait until fractures happen before treatment, physicians will continue to see even more fractures, limitations, and more expensive health care costs.

Specific prevention should begin by age 35 if you have more than 2 of the risk factors for osteoporosis. If you have more than 3 risk factors, then you may consider starting earlier. Stage 1 is the time when there is the greatest chance to actually prevent

the progress of osteoporosis. It is best not to wait until osteoporosis is easily diagnosed even by the newer more sensitive
tests available.

Rule 1: Remove any risk factors possible.

You can make a significant improvement in the prevention
and treatment of osteoporosis by being aware of your own set of
risk factors. Some of these cannot be changed, such as race, sex,
and family history. Yet, some risk factors are quite changeable!

Risk factors which you can change at this stage of prevention of osteoporosis include lack of regular exercise program,
effects of early menopause, cigarette smoking, heavy alcohol
use, certain medications, certain medical problems, and low
calcium in the diet. Injuries and falls should always be prevented, but this becomes much more important in later stages
of osteoporosis when bones become less strong. This is discussed in Chapter Five.

Regular Exercise Is the Key

Check with your physician before you begin any exercise
program. In preventing osteoporosis, you should have a regular
exercise program including a weight-bearing activity. The exact
amount of exercise needed is not known. We suggest regular exercise such as bicycle riding, walking, or running several times
a week for 30 to 40 minutes each session. Weight-bearing activities are some of the strongest natural stimulations for stronger
bones. We are convinced of the importance of regular exercise
in the treatment of osteoporosis, especially when we see the results in even the most severe patients.

In addition to your regular exercise program for osteoporosis prevention and treatment, you need to do exercises to
strengthen the muscles of the back. This may surprise you since
the back is often a source of severe pain. However, there is more
evidence than ever that the patients who improve the most are
those who are able to begin and maintain a regular back exercise
program. Research has shown that the stronger the back muscles
are, the denser the bones in the spine will be. Posture is also improved with exercise. This helps to prevent becoming stooped.

Strong back muscles can only be developed by exercise. Swimming is an excellent exercise but this sport often becomes inconvenient and is not continued regularly. In our clinic, we teach a simple modification of back exercises. If these are performed regularly and properly, a very adequate level of exercise can be maintained at home. These exercises can build needed muscle strength for the back. It has been shown that when the bones in the back are harder, the back muscles are stronger. The goal of these exercises is to make the back muscles strong and flexible.

The simple exercises we recommend in Chapter Seven can be performed easily at home by most people. Check with your physician before beginning any exercise program. Begin very slowly. Because of pain, it may be necessary to begin with only one of the first exercise each day. Gradually increase the number of exercises until you can perform 1 of each exercise every day. Then begin to do 1 of each exercise 2 times a day. Many people find it easiest to do their exercises when they arise in the morning and before they retire at night.

If you have pain, it would be helpful to apply moist heat before you exercise. There are several ways to apply moist heat. Most people find it easiest to put a chair or stool (with rubber tips on the legs for safety) in the shower. Let the warm water hit the back for about 10 minutes. Then do the exercises. Other ways to apply moist heat to the back would be to use a warm bath, warm moist towels, or a whirlpool. Dry or moist heating pads may work as well after you have improved, but may be less effective at first. Choose a method of moist heat which you feel is easiest and most effective for you. Treatments may last about 10 to 20 minutes. The muscles of the back are less tight and exercises are usually easier after moist heat. As you improve, you may find it less important before each exercise session. Then you can use moist heat only as needed for relief of discomfort.

Many osteoporosis patients ask about the usage of pain-relief creams and ointments found in most drugstores. We find that if these creams are appropriately used according to the package directions and IF they do bring some relief to the patient's condition, then this is an acceptable form of treatment.

Exercises to improve your posture can be performed daily while you work, watch television, read, or perform other duties. Being aware of your daily posture is important in keeping back muscles strong and the spine straight. Avoid sitting slumped in a chair or standing in a slouched position. This causes high amounts of stress on the bones of the spine and more strain on the muscles of the back. When sitting, the chair should be firm. Your lower back should be supported by the back of the chair. Try to keep your feet flat on the floor. When standing, your abdominal muscles should be tight and shoulders should be held back. Strong abdominal muscles are important.

Overtraining can be harmful.

Can you get too much exercise? It seems now that for the problem of osteoporosis, the answer is yes in some cases. As we have discussed previously, women who engage in severe physical training such as prolonged, long distance running may develop less regular menstrual periods. Overtraining can cause a temporary change in hormone levels that can result in menstrual changes and in osteoporosis. We recommend that physical training be adjusted or other treatment be added to prevent fractures in this situation.

Correcting the Effects of Early Menopause in Women

There is a much higher risk of osteoporosis after menopause in women. There is more risk if your menstrual period stops before the usual age of 45 to 55, and the risk is higher if you have had both ovaries removed by surgery before menopause. In most people, this higher risk factor can be decreased greatly by taking estrogen, which replaces the usual natural secretion of this hormone by the ovaries. But there are some potential dangers as will be discussed later in this chapter.

Estrogen is vital.

It is now well established that estrogen treatment within the first few years of menopause in women can delay or prevent the progress of osteoporosis. Once bone has been lost and osteoporosis happens, then the body is very limited in its ability to actually replace the bone. Since estrogen is a medication that clearly delays the progress of the loss of bone, researchers would consider the use of estrogens in women who have an early natural menopause or surgical menopause in the hope that bone loss would be prevented.

The most commonly used form of estrogen is conjugated equine estrogen which is available only with a physician's prescription. A few common names of estrogen are included in Table 7.

The dose of estrogen that most researchers suggest is needed to be effective in osteoporosis is the equivalent of 0.625 mg conjugated estrogen daily. This dosage is usually given for 21 to 25 days each month beginning on the first day of each month. The later days of the month no estrogens are taken.

Some physicians add another female hormone in the last seven days of the third week each month. These hormones are called progestins. The progestins are used to lessen the risk of excessive growth of the lining of the uterus. It is thought that progestins might decrease the risk of cancer of the uterus. (As will be discussed, this risk can be managed.)

The use of progestins causes a risk of higher cholesterol and triglycerides in the blood that might increase the risk of coronary artery disease and heart attack. Therefore, until further information is available, some physicians continue estrogen for 21 days each month without progestins. Ask your physician for the best advice in your own case.

If your menopause was natural (without surgery), then you may have bleeding from the vagina after you begin estrogen treatment. By taking estrogen, the uterus is stimulated as it was before menopause. The bleeding may be regular as in a

TABLE 7
Common Estrogen Supplements

Conjugated estrogen tablets	Estraderm transdermal system
Coated conjugated estrogen tablets	Ogen tablets
	Estrace tablets
Estrogen tablets	Estrovis tablets
Premarin tablets	Aygestin tablets
Estratab tablets	

typical menstrual period or it may be spotty. Because there are other serious causes of bleeding (including cancer), it is extremely important for each woman to see her gynecologist or other physician at least once or twice a year. A sample may be taken from the lining of the uterus (different from a pap smear, called endometrial biopsy) to be sure that no other abnormal causes of bleeding are present. This can usually be done conveniently and safely in your physician's office.

Since estrogens were first used for the treatment of osteoporosis, there has been a concern that their use might increase the risk of cancer of the uterus. There is some increased risk, but it can be managed in most cases if low doses of estrogen are used and if regular physician follow-up is continued. No change in the length of life has been found due to such cancers in women who take estrogens after menopause for osteoporosis. The higher risk for cancer of the uterus can be managed by routine examinations by your physician at six-month intervals. If a cancer is found, it is usually discovered in the very early stages and treated easily and effectively.

There have been some suggestions that estrogens might increase the chance of breast cancer in women. Certain women should not take estrogens because of an already higher risk of breast cancer. This might include women who already have had breast cancer and women who have a family history of breast cancer. Regular self-examination, mammogram, and check-ups with your physician should be continued for all women. Your physician can advise you for your particular situation.

Another factor to consider is that estrogen treatment has a beneficial effect on health by lowering the chance of coronary heart disease by as much as 50 percent. Several research teams have found that the overall death rate from every cause is the same or lower in women who use estrogens after menopause. This research, plus newer information about the risk of serious limitation and death from fractures of the hip and other bones, makes estrogen treatment seem more reasonable. If these guidelines are followed with physician advice and follow-up, you can have peace of mind knowing that a worthwhile treatment for osteoporosis can be taken with reasonable safety.

If you have had a hysterectomy, you should not have bleeding from the vagina due to estrogen treatment. The estrogen is taken in the same doses, the equivalent of 0.625 mg conjugated estrogen, daily. You would not need to have the regular yearly test of a sample from the lining of the uterus. But it is still a good idea to have your regular exam by your physician for routine health maintenance, including a pelvic examination.

There is no exact answer available as to how long estrogens should be taken. It is generally believed that calcium supplements or higher calcium in the diet combined with estrogen may make the estrogen treatment more effective in osteoporosis prevention.

Some researchers feel that after 15 or more years following menopause, the lack of estrogen becomes less important for osteoporosis. At this point, other treatments become more important.

It is important for you to be sure that it is safe to take estrogens other than the specific risks already discussed. There are certain other medical problems that can make a person have a higher chance of side effects. These include previous blood clots (thrombophlebitis), heart attack (myocardial infarction), blood clot in the lung (pulmonary embolus), and severe headaches. Because these problems can be very serious, you should discuss your situation with your physician before you begin estrogen treatment. You need to keep in mind that you are trying to prevent the potentially crippling and devastating problem of osteoporosis, but you must do it safely. This is possible with a reasonable amount of care. This does not need to be very time-consuming or expensive.

Benefits may outweigh the risks.

You may consider the overall benefits and risks when deciding whether or not to take estrogens. Recent research has shown that the benefits of estrogen treatment in preventing fractures of the hips and other bones after menopause seem to outweigh the risks in many, but not all, women. Remember, there is a risk of serious limitation when a fracture of the hip or other bone occurs. But in some women, estrogen treatment may not be worth the risks. Ask your physician to help decide what is best for your situation.

Stop Cigarette Smoking

Smoking may double your risk of getting osteoporosis as well as increase your chances for heart disease, stroke, cancer, and lung diseases. Knowing these facts, you should make a concerted effort to stop smoking.

You can call your local chapter of the American Lung Association for information on stop-smoking clinics or your physician may recommend such treatments as hypnosis or the prescription nicotine patch. Most of our patients who use the patch are successful in kicking this deadly habit. Stopping any habit is not easy, but the rewards from quitting smoking far outweigh the first few difficult days. If you need help in stopping smoking, seek assistance from a qualified, reputable smoking clinic or your physician.

Stop Heavy Alcohol Use

Alcohol has recently been seen as a contributing cause in osteoporosis in some people—men as well as women. The disease is usually found in those people who have had a heavy alcohol intake for a number of years. These patients may feel pain in the back and may have fractures as in other causes of osteoporosis. Those affected are often as young as age 30 to 40, younger than usual for fractures from most other causes of osteoporosis.

If you are a heavy alcohol drinker, check with support groups in your community such as Alcoholics Anonymous for information in getting rid of this drug. We recommend that patients who can tolerate alcohol, limit the alcohol intake to $1/2$ to 1 oz. of distilled liquor or $1/2$ bottle of wine or 12 to 24 oz. of beer daily or less. Small amounts of alcohol are acceptable in cooking as most of the alcohol evaporates.

Be Aware of Certain Medications

Some medications taken for other medical problems can increase the risk of developing osteoporosis. One of the most common is the group of cortisone-like drugs. Remember that all of these related drugs increase the risk of osteoporosis. There are many different names and forms of cortisone. These drugs may be necessary to control other diseases.

If it is necessary to take one of this group of medications, always try to take the lowest possible dose for the shortest length of time recommended by your physician. Also be sure that you are following the other ways to prevent osteoporosis. If this is done, these cortisone-like drugs can be taken with the least amount of added risk for osteoporosis.

Antacids are very commonly advertised and widely used tablets or liquids taken to neutralize stomach acid, treat heartburn and indigestion, treat ulcers in the stomach or duodenum, and to treat other problems. Many of these antacids contain aluminum. If taken regularly, this can result in an excessive loss of calcium from the body. Calcium is removed from the bones in the body's attempt to make up for the extra calcium loss. This makes it harder for the body to form new bone. A higher intake of calcium in the diet may offset this extra calcium loss. Be aware of this possibility and avoid frequent high doses of antacids containing aluminum.

Thyroid medication is used to treat those people who for many different reasons may have less than normal levels of thyroid hormone in their body. If an excessive amount of thyroid medication is present, osteoporosis and fractures can occur. This would be similar to the problem of an overactive thyroid gland which produces too much thyroid hormone. Recent research suggests that even normal and correct amounts of thyroid medication given to patients may at times result in osteoporosis. In these cases, prevention might include decreasing the dose of thyroid medication as well as the other prevention for osteoporosis. If the patient has osteoporosis, treatment should include decreasing the dose of thyroid medication and following the guidelines for treatment outlined in Chapter Five. Let your physician guide you in making these changes should you need thyroid medication.

Other Medical Problems

For reasons that are not clear, certain medical problems seem to increase the chance of osteoporosis. These problems are discussed in Chapter Two. If you have one of these problems, it will be important to have the best possible control and treatment. Your physician can help you control these problems which can accelerate osteoporosis:

- Rheumatoid arthritis
- Diabetes mellitus
- Emphysema and chronic bronchitis
- Certain types of surgery on the stomach, especially removal of part of the stomach
- Other uncommon medical problems

Correct Low Calcium in Diet

Research suggests that increasing the amount of calcium in a diet might slow osteoporosis in women. But it is very difficult to do scientific experiments in humans for this type of diet. High-calcium diets over a lifetime, especially in the developing years, seem more likely to increase the amount of bone formed as the skeleton matures. This would allow more bone to be present before the process of osteoporosis begins. The idea is to build the maximum bone strength before osteoporosis slowly decreases the amount of bone present. A careful diet for calcium intake should begin in childhood. The average intake of calcium in the United States has been estimated to be 450 to 550 mg each day, but the adult requirement for calcium is 1000 mg each day.

To help prevent osteoporosis, the recommended calcium intake for women before menopause is 1000 mg daily. It is reasonable to have similar recommendations for men, with particular emphasis on adequate calcium intake after age 50. The recommended intake of calcium for children is 800 mg daily with 1200 mg daily for teenagers. The calcium intake for women who are pregnant and for nursing mothers is 1200 mg daily (see Table 5).

Adequate calcium intake can be assured by taking calcium in the diet or by taking supplements of calcium. Diet calcium can be increased easily with a few suggestions. Be sure to include 3 or 4 servings of calcium-rich foods each day in your diet. One serving of milk and dairy products with three meals each day could give a majority of your daily calcium needs. Just 2 glasses of skim milk along with 1 cup of nonfat yogurt would complete the 1000 mg you need each day. Use the chart to estimate daily intake, then add a calcium supplement if necessary.

If you are trying to limit your daily caloric intake to lose weight or to avoid gaining weight, it is not necessary to completely eliminate dairy products from your diet. You may want to choose low-fat skim milk products. These products usually offer the same calcium benefits without the higher calories. Many newer products including low-fat cheese slices and low-fat yogurt are now available as well as high calcium low-fat hot chocolate mixes.

Vitamin D is needed by the body to help the absorption of calcium. Sun exposure allows the body to make vitamin D. Drinking vitamin D-fortified milk can also supply the body's needs. Certain foods are richer in vitamin D than others (see Table 8, p. 63).

Dieticians offer a few other suggestions to help in choosing foods best for the body's calcium needs. High amounts of fat and protein in the diet can interfere with calcium absorption. This would suggest that excessive fatty foods be avoided, especially if taken at the same time as calcium-rich foods or calcium supplements.

Certain foods can increase the intake of phosphates (especially common in soft drinks and many convenience foods). If continued, this could result in more loss of calcium from the body because of the way the body manages phosphorus. Moderate amounts of such foods in the diet seem to be acceptable.

Some foods that contain calcium such as vegetables may also contain oxalate. Green leafy vegetables such as spinach contain oxalate. This oxalate may decrease the body's absorption of the calcium in this product. In such cases, even though the food may contain calcium, it may not be as available to the body as the calcium in other foods. Knowledge of this fact can allow you to include other sources of calcium as well.

Some studies have found evidence that high amounts of caffeine in the diet might increase calcium loss. Caffeine is present in many drinks including coffee, colas, and other soft drinks. It would be reasonable to avoid excessive intake until further knowledge of caffeine in osteoporosis is available.

In addition to diet calcium, adequate calcium intake can be assured by taking supplements of calcium. A simple way to assure enough calcium is to take tablets or capsules. These supplements usually have no calories, which helps those who are trying to lose weight. Keep in mind that different forms of calcium are available.

The least expensive form of calcium can be as effective as the higher priced tablets and capsules as long as the proper amount of calcium is contained in the product. Just be sure that you take the correct total amount of calcium. This information should be available on the package or bottle label.

Each form of calcium may have different amounts of calcium actually available to your body. Calcium carbonate or oyster shell are the common forms of calcium that have the highest percent of calcium available for your body to absorb and use for bone formation. About 40 percent of calcium carbonate or oyster shell is available as calcium for your body to absorb. This means that if a tablet contains 500 mg of calcium carbonate or oyster shell then it will give your body about 200 mg of calcium available for absorption.

Calcium lactate has less actual calcium available for the body to absorb. A tablet which contains 650 mg calcium will have about 84.5 mg available to your body. If you have a consistently lower than recommended calcium intake, you should consider adding more calcium such as dairy products to your diet. Or, consider a calcium supplement.

The main side effect from taking too much calcium is the risk of development of kidney stones. If you have had a kidney stone, you should definitely ask your physician before you begin a higher calcium intake. Then you can decide whether the benefits would be worth the risks. If it is important in your case that calcium be used, then urine tests and other studies are available which can help to tell whether it would be safe for you to continue the higher calcium intake.

Remember that vitamin D increases the body's absorption of calcium. If excess vitamin D is taken (especially in high doses) along with calcium, it can cause more calcium to be absorbed. This can cause high levels of calcium in the blood which can result in nausea, constipation, and serious illness. Careful use of vitamin D is needed. This is discussed in Chapter Five. In Stage 1, Prevention, vitamin D intake can be limited to the recommended daily requirement for adults of 200 units and for children, 400 units.

A particular calcium supplement may cause nausea, may be difficult for you to swallow, or may cause other unwanted side effects for you. Choose the one that is most convenient for you and causes no side effects.

=============== SUMMARY ===============

STAGE 1: Prevention: Before Osteoporosis Is Detectable

1. Remove any risk factors present.
2. Begin a regular exercise program.
3. After menopause in women, consider adding estrogen on the advice of your physician.
4. Stop cigarettes.
5. Avoid heavy alcohol intake.
6. Limit those medications which increase the chance of osteoporosis.
7. Treat those other medical problems which contribute to osteoporosis.
8. For osteoporosis prevention, adults need 1000 mg calcium daily in the diet and calcium supplements.

CHAPTER FIVE

A Treatment Plan for Osteoporosis

As stated previously, osteoporosis has no known cure. While it is reasonable that prevention measures would be the most appropriate way to halt or slow the progress of the disease, there are methods of treatment that can prove beneficial to the osteoporosis patient.

Prevention measures must begin in childhood, adolescence, and young adulthood to reap the greatest benefits. As discussed in Chapter Four, osteoporosis occurs sometime after a person has reached maturity. Aggressive measures for prevention taken at Stage 1 can result in diminishing the chances of developing osteoporosis and the debilitating fractures.

Stage 2:
Osteoporosis Becomes Detectable

Stage 2 osteoporosis usually begins from age 35 or older. If there are many risk factors present, this stage can begin even earlier. At this point, the gradual decrease in bone formation described in Stage 1 has been taking place, usually for years. In addition, the process of bone removal has continued. Very slowly the total amount of bone and the density of bone has decreased. The bones are still strong enough so that no unusual fractures occur. This is before any symptoms of pain or fractures occur but years after the prevention stage discussed in Chapter Four. The osteoporosis eventually becomes detectable by routine X-rays such as a chest X-ray or other X-rays. It is also possible to detect osteoporosis by a bone density screening test as described in Chapter Four. At this time, these tests are the most sensitive and easily available methods to tell if you have osteoporosis. Chapter Three discusses the tests currently available and suggests some guidelines for deciding whether you might want to consider proceeding with testing.

If osteoporosis is detected by any of these tests, but no fractures have occurred, it is reasonable to take action for treatment of the osteoporosis. Hopefully, immediate action through treatment will prevent fractures. Several rules are important to follow.

Rule 1: Remove any risk factors possible.

You can still delay the progress of osteoporosis at this point. A person in Stage 2 should try to remove all possible risk factors just as in Stage 1, Chapter Four.

Rule 2: Decide if other medications should be used.

Estrogen Treatment

Estrogen treatment should be strongly considered at Stage 2 in women who have reached menopause because the osteoporosis is already definitely established. Remember that estrogens are most effective when used early in osteoporosis. Talk to your physician. Review the discussion in Chapter Three about estrogen treatment. If there are no reasons to avoid estrogens in your case, then it is usually strongly recommended.

Vitamin D Is Recommended

One of the uses of vitamin D by the body is to help absorb calcium from the intestine. Some osteoporosis patients have a lower level of vitamin D and a less effective absorption of calcium from the intestine. Vitamin D is either made in the body from exposure to sunlight or is taken through foods.

This vitamin is recommended as medication in order to increase the body's absorption of calcium, increasing the amount of calcium available to the body for bone formation. Unfortunately, there has been little convincing proof that adding very high doses of vitamin D helps prevent fractures or delays osteoporosis. There may be a beneficial effect, but it has not been shown yet. Researchers have found that vitamin D alone does not prevent bone loss caused by the loss of estrogens at menopause. It is therefore not an alternative to estrogen treatment. If you do not have an adequate amount of vitamin D in your diet, and you do not receive very much sunlight exposure, then vitamin D supplementation is definitely needed.

People who spend most of their time indoors are especially at risk for lack of vitamin D. The standard recommended intake of vitamin D is 300 to 400 units daily. To increase absorption of calcium from the intestine, vitamin D intake can be increased up to 800 units daily, which can be taken in through food in the diet or as a supplement. Foods containing vitamin D are listed in the table. Some of the choices available for vitamin D supplements which are available at drug stores or health food stores are listed on the next page.

Very high doses of vitamin D (above 800 units daily) can raise the calcium levels in the blood higher than normal and result in illness. These higher doses should be prescribed and monitored by your physician. Vitamin D in lower doses can be purchased at pharmacies and health food stores or as prescribed by your physician.

Tables 8 and 9 show some common sources of vitamin D in foods and supplements.

Vitamin D Supplements

Calciferol	Higher doses by prescription
Ergocalciferol	Lower doses over the counter
Vitamin D2	At drugstores or health food stores

Stage 3:
Osteoporosis with Fractures

Stage 3 usually happens between ages 55 to 70, but can begin earlier, especially if other problems are present such as

TABLE 8
Some Sources of Vitamin D in Foods

Food	Serving Size	Vitamin D (IU)
Cereals		
Bran Flakes	¾ cup	100
Raisin Bran	¾ cup	100
Eel, smoked	3 ½ oz.	6400
Egg	1 medium	27
Egg substitute	¼ cup	26
Margarine	1 Tablespoon	45
Sardines, canned in oil	3 ½ oz.	300
Salmon (Atlantic), canned	3 ½ oz.	500
Milk, fortified	1 cup	100
Milk, evaporated, canned	½ cup	88

early menopause, certain medications, heavy alcohol use, or excessive physical training. In most cases, osteoporosis has been present for a number of years but has gone undetected.

At Stage 3, enough loss of bone density and strength occurs that an accident results in fracture. The accident may be severe enough to cause a fracture under normal circumstances, such as a fall or an auto collision. Or, the accident may be quite minor, such as a stumble. Fractures may occur in the spine, the hip, the wrists, or in other bones. As Stage 3 advances, less

TABLE 9
Calcium with Vitamin D Supplements

Name	Form of Calcium	Actual Amount of Calcium Available	Amount of Vitamin D
Calcet tablets	calcium lactate	240 mg/tablet	100 IU
	calcium gluconate	240 mg/tablet	
	calcium carbonate	152 mg/tablet	
Dical-D capsules	calcium diphosphonate	3 capsules: 350 mg	3 capsules: 399 IU
Dical-D wafers	calcium diphosphonate	2 wafers: 464 mg	2 wafers: 400 IU
Os-Cal 250 tablets	oyster shell	250 mg/tablet	125 IU

injury is required to cause a fracture. Eventually, even normal daily activities such as walking or lifting may cause a fracture.

Rule 1: Fractures require medical attention.

When a hip, wrist, or other bone is fractured, proper care by an orthopedist is necessary. This may or may not involve an operation depending on the severity of the fracture. For hip fractures, the strongest advantage of an operation is that it allows the patient to begin walking much earlier. A patient may be in the hospital for 7 to 10 days and may be able to walk by the time the hospital stay is over. Without the operation, it may require six weeks or more of bedrest and then very slow progress in beginning to walk again. Such a long time in bed is dangerous for many reasons. The extended bedrest can increase the chances of blood clot formation in the legs and pelvis, resulting in blood clots moving to the lungs and risk of death. This period of inactivity also increases the development of osteoporosis which is the basic problem we are trying to solve!

In a fracture of the vertebral body in the spine, which usually involves the middle or lower back, the pain may be severe. It often comes on suddenly and may last 3 to 6 weeks.

A person may feel pain in the middle of the back after lifting. It can also happen after bending or stooping. Some people first notice the discomfort upon arising in the morning. The pain can result from a fracture of the thoracic or the lumbar part of the spine. The pain is usually most severe at first and can last a few days up to a few weeks. Usually after a few weeks, the discomfort begins to subside. Bedrest is often needed at first to relieve the pain. Sitting and standing usually make the pain worse. After it has decreased, it is usually possible to gradually begin sitting. Standing and walking can be attempted next. It is very important to follow the guidelines your physician sets for a gradual increase in activity. Your physician can make sure no other problems are present that would need treatment. Some serious diseases can cause fractures in the spine and may require specific treatment. As the pain eases, activity can usually be gradually increased if pain does not increase with the activity.

During the period of severe pain, medications are usually needed. The pain is often so severe that it is difficult to sleep. Some pain relievers are available over-the-counter such as ibuprofen (Advil). If the pain is not able to be controlled by these medications, we may use another pain medication such as propoxyphene (Darvon) alone or combined with acetaminophen (Darvocet) or codeine with acetaminophen. These pain relievers require a prescription and should be used very carefully. Use these prescription medications only during the days and nights that the pain is severe, then change to Advil or another pain reliever as soon as you feel some relief.

Some patients with fractures may need to be admitted to a hospital to relieve the pain. In the hospital or physician's office, a patient may be seen by a physical therapist to help begin gradual increase in activity and exercise.

Pain Control for Osteoporosis

Nonprescription	Prescription
Ibuprofen (Advil)	Propoxyphene (Darvon)
Acetaminophen	Codeine
Aspirin	

Gradually Add Exercise

Once the severe pain associated with Stage 3 has improved, the use of pain medicine should be avoided as much as possible. As activities such as sitting, standing, and walking are possible, an exercise program can be added with proper instruction and supervision as described on page 79. At Stage 3, the patient may use a brace or support for the spine. The brace should be used for as short a period as possible because these supports do not help the body increase the strength of the muscles of the back. The use of a brace might encourage the muscles of the back to be less strong if used over a long period of time. Supports can be used if it becomes necessary to increase a person's activity faster than the pain allows.

In our clinic, we generally have not found braces to be very useful at this point. We have found that patients often do not like to use braces because they are frequently heavy, hot, and expensive.

The importance of an exercise program cannot be emphasized enough. We discuss regular exercise again and again with our patients so that this major part of the treatment is understood and followed.

Rule 2: Remove all risk factors possible.

Once the fracture has healed, begin to remove the risk factors as described in Chapter Four. It is never too late to begin actions which might delay the further loss of bone. Each risk factor that can be eliminated will help to decrease the chance of the next fracture. Remember, these fractures will heal. Then it is time to do everything possible to stop fractures in the future.

Prevention of accidents and falls becomes more important in Stage 3. Since bone strength has been lost, less injury than usual can result in fractures. It is especially important at this point to review the discussion of the safe living chart in Chapter Three to learn how to make the patient's environment as safe as possible. Use the checklist to be sure there will be no accidents that could have been prevented.

Rule 3: Medications to consider.

Calcium, Vitamin D, Estrogens

Medications to include at Stage 3 include calcium supplements, approximately 1500 mg per day, and vitamin D, up to 800 units daily if the patient's vitamin intake or sun exposure is not adequate. Vitamin D supplements would apply especially to people who are severely restricted in activity such as those patients in nursing homes. Vitamin D can be purchased at health food stores or can be obtained from your pharmacy with a prescription.

If Stage 3 occurs within a few years of menopause, estrogen treatment should be considered. If menopause was more than 20 years earlier, then estrogen may still help but the evidence is not as clear yet. Some researchers would suggest adding estrogens up to age 75 depending on your individual situation. If there is no other problem present which could make the use of estrogens unsafe, then you may consider the use of this medication with the advice of your physician. It may be a number of years before this question is finally answered. Discuss this matter with your physician for the best answer in your situation. Read the discussion of estrogen treatment on pages 50–54.

Fluoride

A medicine that can be used but is not yet approved by the Food and Drug Administration is fluoride. Fluoride has been used for years in osteoporosis since it was noticed that the population in areas with higher fluoride content in their drinking water have fewer fractures from osteoporosis. It is thought that fluoride increases bone formation and bone density. It is important to have adequate calcium intake in your diet or to take calcium supplements along with the fluoride. Some researchers have found an increase in the bone density in patients who took fluoride. It usually takes 1 to 2 years of treatment to show a response in bone. Some researchers have found 4 to 5 years of treatment to be more effective.

Although fluoride increases the bone density, it has not always been shown to actually lower the number of fractures in osteoporosis and is not routinely used. Higher doses of fluoride may cause nausea, diarrhea, and acute attacks of pain in the joints and bones. Tests are continuing at this time to try to find out just how effective fluoride is and the lowest dose needed for protection in osteoporosis with the least side effects. Until these tests are completed, fluoride treatment may be considered for more severe osteoporosis, but only under the careful directions of your physician. The cost varies but is generally $10 to $20 per month depending on the dose.

Calcitonin

Calcitonin is a hormone which is normally made in the body. One of its actions is to lower the activity of the cells which remove calcium from bones. Calcitonin was tried in osteoporosis patients because it appears that some cases of osteoporosis may be caused by too rapid removal of bone. Some tests have shown that there is an increase in bone density in women with osteoporosis after being treated with calcitonin. It is not definite that calcitonin also prevents fractures although it seems reasonable to expect this effect. Testing in a number of centers is now being done to answer this question. The more severe the osteoporosis, the more reasonable it would be to consider treatment with calcitonin. Your physician can help you decide if it would be worthwhile.

Calcitonin is not absorbed if taken by mouth. Therefore, the medication must be given by injection. The usual recommended dose is given two times weekly up to a daily injection. The injections may be given in the muscle of the arm or leg. The cost of the medicine and syringes for three injections weekly would be $60 to $130 per month. Side effects such as nausea and rashes may occur but are generally not a major problem in most patients. Brand names for calcitonin are Calcimar and Cibacalcin.

There are other medications that are used to treat osteoporosis, especially if other treatment has not been successful. One group of medicines that is being used can slow the removal of bone but still allows for bone formation. One that is used now is etidronate (Didronel), but must be given with close supervision by your physician. Others are being developed and will be available in the next few years.

Stage 4:
Osteoporosis with Chronic
Pain and Deformity

Stage 4 may happen from age 55. At this time, osteoporosis gradually becomes severe enough so that even minor amounts of physical stress or injury cause fractures. These fractures happen most commonly in the vertebral bodies of the middle or the lower back. The vertebral body becomes shorter. This stage may cause a loss of height and a stooped posture which has become well known over the past few years with osteoporosis patients. There is often severe pain in the middle and lower back which seems unending. Any bone may become fractured. At Stage 4, a person may have a fracture of a rib occur through minor impact or even through their usual daily activity. One patient suffered a rib fracture during a strong hug from her son returning home from the Navy.

Rule 1: Fractures require medical attention.

The treatment for Stage 4 is similar to Stage 3 if a fracture occurs. As soon as the acute fracture heals adequately, an increase in activity and an exercise program should begin as on pages 81–98. At Stage 4, many patients find it hard to understand how exercise will help. There must be strong encouragement at this time. People who are totally disabled by pain are later able to resume most of their activities if they are able to continue a regular program of exercise and other treatment. Braces may be used at Stage 4 but should be avoided when possible because they do not encourage the strengthening of back muscles, although they do allow more activity in some cases.

Rule 2: Remove any risk factors possible.

It is important to remove all possible risk factors to prevent future osteoporosis as described in Chapter Three.

Rule 3: Medications are necessary for Stage 4.

Medications used at this stage are the same as in earlier stages including calcium and vitamin D. There is no definite proof that the estrogens will cause fewer fractures if given at this stage, but it is possible that the osteoporosis may be delayed. There is simply not enough information yet to make a definite recommendation on the use of estrogens in this stage. If there is no other problem present which could make the use of estrogens unsafe, then you can consider this medication with the advice of your physician. At Stage 4, the patient should consider other medications. The benefits of preventing more fractures are even more important. These other medications (discussed on page 65) are usually tolerated with few side effects. These medications should definitely be taken under the supervision of a physician. At Stage 4, the use of several different medications should be considered that might help without causing serious side effects.

This program will work!

Encouragement is required for the osteoporosis patient at Stage 4. Severe pain has usually been present for some time that may lead to discouragement, depression, and thoughts of suicide. A person at this point must understand that the program outlined can and does work. Progress may first be slow but usually improvement is noted after a few weeks to several months. Patients commonly become discouraged over slow progress. In a large majority of patients, there is better control of pain and improved activity once they begin the outlined program of treatment. Patients with osteoporosis so severe that proper treatment and supervision does not result in some improvement are unusual. The use of pain medicines at this time may be needed. We limit the use of narcotics, which usually do not give complete relief and may become habit-forming. Other methods of chronic pain control may be useful at Stage 4 including certain medications and evaluation in a pain clinic. Pain clinics attempt to help a person control and live with the pain more comfortably. In such a clinic all aspects of pain from its cause to its management and control are studied. Many different methods may be used to help control pain and a person's response to pain. Such a clinic requires more time and expense but is often worthwhile for control of pain and return of the patient to activity.

SUMMARY

STAGE 2: Osteoporosis Becomes Detectable.
1. Remove risk factors present as in Stage 1.
2. Begin a regular exercise program.
3. Consider adding estrogen in women after menopause on the advice of your physician.

4. Be sure of 1500 mg of calcium daily and adequate vitamin D intake.

STAGE 3: Osteoporosis Results in Fractures.

1. Treat the acute fracture as directed by your physician.
2. Begin your regular exercise program as soon as it becomes possible.
3. Remove risk factors as in Stage 1.
4. Be sure of 1500 mg of calcium daily and adequate vitamin D intake.
5. Consider other medications as discussed plus estrogen in women on the advice of your physician.

STAGE 4: Osteoporosis with Chronic Pain and Deformity.

1. Treat the fracture if present as directed by your physician.
2. Begin a regular exercise program as soon as it becomes possible.
3. Remove risk factors as in Stage 1.
4. Be sure of 1500 mg calcium daily and adequate vitamin D intake.
5. Consider other medications as discussed plus estrogen in women on the advice of your physician.
6. Realize that encouragement and positive thinking are important to your overall well-being.

CHAPTER SIX

Setting the Stage:
Infants, Children, Teenagers

Osteoporosis does not have to follow generation after generation in families leaving its debilitating mark of pain and disfigurement. Even though having a family member with osteoporosis increases a person's risk of acquiring osteoporosis, preventive measures can be taken.

Calcium needs must be met during pregnancy and breast feeding to provide for both mother and infant. During pregnancy, calcium needs are up from 800 mg to 1200 mg. Most of this need for calcium occurs during the last 2 to 3 months of pregnancy coinciding with calcification of the fetal skeleton. Calcium is transferred from the mother's bones to the fetus, justifying the increased need throughout pregnancy.

Adequate calcium during pregnancy and breast feeding is needed for bone and tooth development of the baby and prevents loss of calcium from the mother's bones during breast feeding. Studies indicate that low calcium intakes during pregnancy (below 350 mg) are associated with an increased incidence of pregnancy-induced hypertension (eclampsia). Some evidence indicates that increased calcium intake during pregnancy lowers blood pressure in healthy pregnant women.

With prevention of osteoporosis in later life as the goal, adults need to be aware of specific steps that can be taken to

72

protect infants, children, and teenagers from the disease in the future, many years before the real stages of osteoporosis set in.

Infants

At birth, the bones have less calcium content than at other times of life. Over the first year, this bone calcium content increases faster than at any period of time, especially during periods of rapid growth.

For the nursing mother, breast milk contains about 300 mg calcium per liter. The infant retains about two thirds of this amount of calcium. Cow's milk formulas contain about 600 to 700 mg of calcium per liter; however, the infant only retains 25 to 30 percent of this amount. The infant's needs can be adequately met with either form of feeding. (See Dietary Allowance Chart for Calcium on p. 34.) A maternal diet deficient in calcium has little influence over the calcium content of the breast milk due to the regulation of the mother's own calcium stores. If calcium and phosphorus are deficient in the mother's diet, these minerals are removed from her bone stores to form milk.

From birth to age 2 the bones are in a rapid phase of active growth characterized by an increase in bone length. Width shaping of the bones also occurs at this time. The necessary nutrients during this development for healthy bones and teeth are calcium, phosphorus, protein, magnesium, fluoride, and vitamins A, C, and D. Most infants receive these important nutrients from breast milk or fortified formulas. Infants who are not breast-fed and are allergic to cow's milk formula can still receive adequate calcium in the available soy formulas.

Children

Calcium retention slows down in the childhood years. Growing children still need 2 to 4 times as much calcium per body weight as adults. One study showed that women who drank milk every meal during childhood and adolescence had significantly higher bone density than women who drank milk less frequently. Milk drinking is not only necessary for growth and development, but to assure an optimal peak of bone mass for later years.

Children must receive the Recommended Daily Allowance of calcium each day. Exercises, especially those that involve movement and pull on the bones, stimulate the growth and increase the density of the bones. Weight-bearing exercises such as walking, cycling, climbing stairs, and jumping rope are recommended for children. Most children are assured of adequate exercise through the usual playtime activities.

Although childhood is an extremely important time for building dense bones, many children shun milk for various reasons. Using the calcium chart in Chapter Two, look at some favorite sources of calcium. Working with your child, maintain the proper Recommended Daily Allowance for the specific age group as indicated on the chart on page 34.

A typical day's diet for your child might include 2 cups of milk with 1 oz. of cheese. Part of the milk may be in the form of dessert such as yogurt or pudding, or the cheese might be melted on a favorite vegetable. If your child still shuns milk and milk products, you will need to supplement with powdered skim milk added to foods or with calcium supplements. Use skim or lowfat milk, cheeses, cottage cheese, and yogurt to avoid excess cholesterol and fat in diets. If necessary, supplement your child's diet with calcium tablets.

Lactose is a carbohydrate in milk and milk products that increases calcium absorption. In lactose intolerance, symptoms such as nausea, bloating, and intestinal cramps occur several hours after the ingestion of milk or milk products. If your child has lactose intolerance, he is often at a greater risk of calcium deficiency, and thus, osteoporosis in later years. Often heated milk is tolerated by these individuals. It can be served in hot chocolate, in a cream sauce, cream soup, custard, or pudding. A commercial product called Lactaid® is available in most drugstores. This product can be added to milk to reduce the amount of lactose. Lactaid® contains lactase, an enzyme which breaks down the lactose in milk, thereby eliminating much of the problem for the lactose-intolerant person. If all milk products must be avoided, a calcium supplement is needed.

Vitamin D is also important to calcium absorption and bone mineralization. A deficiency of vitamin D decreases calcium absorption. Adequate exposure to the sun (15 minutes per day) and drinking vitamin D-fortified milk can assure your child the Recommended Daily Allowance.

Teenagers

Teenage girls especially need to be aware that osteoporosis in future years can be prevented. During the teenage years, the bones are developing rapidly. If enough calcium is taken during these years—especially during the late teen years—the chances are that bones will have maximum development and strength.

The teenage years are the time in which the supply of bone is built. The denser the bones become during these years, the longer the density of the bones may last when the process of bone removal begins later in life. The goal should be to build the most dense supply of bones while bone building is already very rapid. This can be achieved if the teenager's diet contains enough of the building blocks needed to form bone. The diet needs to include enough calcium (at least 1200 mg daily) as well as ample protein, vitamins, and minerals.

The total of 1200 mg calcium needed by teenage girls each day may come from diet calcium and calcium supplements.

An accurate way to ensure adequate calcium for teenage girls is to estimate how much calcium is usually consumed in an average day. Working with your teen, list all of the foods for one day using Table 10. Now turn to Table 12 on pages 102 through 116 and find out how much calcium is contained in each food and drink, and fill in the proper totals in the diary. If the total calcium for one average day (or the average of seven days) is less than about 1200 mg, then a calcium supplement should be added to bring the total calcium intake for the day up to 1200 mg.

As important as it is during the teenage years to get enough calcium in the diet, it is also important to establish the habit of taking care of the body. There is a good chance that if a teenage girl understands the need for calcium in her diet and realizes the importance of a proper diet, this may continue for years into her adult life. The habits formed in the teenage years may allow her to continue to build denser bones during the

TABLE 10
Calcium Diary

	Breakfast	Amount of Calcium	Lunch	Amount of Calcium	Dinner	Amount of Calcium	Snacks	Amount of Calcium
Monday								
Tuesday								
Wednesday								
Thursday								
Friday								
Saturday								
Sunday								

After each meal or snack, write down the foods eaten. Go to the table on pp. 102–116 and fill in the amount of calcium for each food and portion. Your daily intake of calcium should meet the standards in Table 5, the Recommended Daily Allowance Chart on page 34. If you find that your diet is low in calcium, make up the difference with calcium supplements.

important adult years and help to prevent osteoporosis. Remember, the greater the amount of bone present at the beginning of osteoporosis, Stage 1, the longer the density of the bones will last.

Educating teenagers about osteoporosis is vital. We have found that once teenage girls learn the facts, most are eager to make the needed additions to their diet to be sure of enough calcium. As our society has become more aware of osteoporosis and the need for prevention, it has become easier for teenagers to get the facts about prevention of the disease. In fact, many public and private schools now include facts on osteoporosis and calcium in the regular curriculum beginning in the 6th and 7th grades.

The word osteoporosis is no longer distant and difficult. We have found that teenagers quickly learn the basics of calcium and diet to help prevent osteoporosis. Teenage boys benefit from the knowledge of diet and calcium as well. Men are also at risk for osteoporosis even though it usually begins at a later age than in women.

A growing concern among teenage girls is weight control. Many adolescents are obsessed with maintaining a low body weight, and a great number of teens frequently diet to avoid gaining extra pounds. Because good sources of calcium such as milk and cheese contain high calories, these foods are often deleted from the weight loss diet. As a result, the total amount of calcium consumed daily may be quite low. Misinformed teens can do great bodily harm by excluding calcium from their diets and may pay the price in later years.

Some understanding assistance from adults in such cases may be useful. Foods such as skim and low-fat milk can be used with meals or for a low-calorie snack. Plain yogurt is not only low in calories, but can be sweetened with fresh fruit for breakfast. And you can add non-fat milk powder to foods such as hot cereals, baked goods, or meat dishes to supplement the calcium intake. If calcium in the diet is consistently low, then add a calcium supplement during dieting.

Exercise is also important during the teenage years. A good exercise program may include running, racquetball, tennis, or other activities that can increase the density of bones, help in weight control, and improve overall fitness. Just as in a healthy, balanced diet, habits formed during the teenage years have a good chance of being continued in later adult life.

We must add a word of caution. Some teenage girls participate in very strenuous training and physical exercise, especially in competitive sports such as running. If training and physical activity is strenuous enough to cause menstrual periods to change or stop, a change in the body's hormone system may have occurred. This problem can be remedied if the level of training is changed temporarily. You should discuss this with your physician as this problem can be treated effectively and may allow for further physical training.

Removing other risk factors for osteoporosis is important in the teenage years. Smoking may double the risk of osteoporosis. If smoking is avoided or stopped during these years there will be added health benefits as well as aiding in the prevention of osteoporosis. Removal of other risk factors as described in Chapter Two is important for all ages, including the teenage years.

Because most teenagers are on busy schedules with school, extra-curricular activities, part-time jobs, and studying, fast foods and convenience foods are used frequently. Be *aware* of the calcium content of these foods.

The complete calcium guide found in Chapter Eight (Table 12) can assist you and your teen in ensuring an adequate calcium intake each day.

SUMMARY

1. Adequate calcium intake is important in all stages of life.
2. Infants, children, and nursing mothers need adequate calcium from their diet or calcium supplement.
3. Teenagers, especially teenage girls, need to know that today's diet can affect their future. 1200 mg of calcium daily is recommended for teenage girls by diet or supplement.
4. Adequate calcium intake can be assured for children and teenagers by being aware of the calcium content of common foods and by the use of calcium supplements.

CHAPTER SEVEN

A Daily
Exercise Program

Exercises are one of the best long-term ways to increase the strength of back and hip muscles; therefore, the importance of a daily exercise program cannot be overestimated as part of managing your osteoporosis. In our clinic we have found that people in all stages of osteoporosis who are able to begin and maintain an adequate exercise program are almost always able to improve. Those people who are not able to begin and maintain a regular exercise program are usually those who still live with tremendous pain from osteoporosis. If you can't do these exercises or you experience pain when you do the exercises, stop and talk to your physician. Then you can find a way to establish the best level of exercise for you.

It usually requires weeks to learn the exercises effectively and to be able to perform the correct number of repetitions twice daily. A commitment on your part to follow through with the program is a must.

Do not be concerned if as you begin you can only do one repetition of the first exercise. You should have no more pain after you finish than when you begin the exercises. If you experience severe pain while exercising, you should stop. After a few days, try two repetitions of one or two exercises. When you have mastered this number, try three or four repetitions, gradually increasing the number of exercises and repetitions. The goal is to perform 10 to 20 repetitions of each exercise two times daily. This is the level that we feel is most useful to maintain the highest level of movement and strength for the back muscles. Remember to do these exercises slowly.

We realize that there will be some days when you do not feel the need for exercise. You may feel uncomfortable or tired. In order to achieve maximum relief from the pain and disfigurement of osteoporosis, you must begin a regular and compulsive program of twice-daily exercise to be done every day— good days and bad days as well.

Beginning a Daily Exercise Program

Exercises are most effective when done properly. You should be instructed by a qualified physical therapist or physician. The following exercises are most effective if performed daily. Check with your physician before you begin any exercise program. Start with one or two repetitions per day and slowly increase. If you have any questions, check with your doctor or physical therapist. If you have pain, stop and talk with your physician before beginning the exercises again.

Neck

These neck exercises improve the mobility and flexibility of the neck. Flexibility is important to help your body perform more effectively. You may sit or stand to do these exercises, whichever is more comfortable for you (see Figure 9).

1. Bend the chin forward to the chest. If you feel stiffness or pain, do not force the movement. Go as far as you can move easily. If pain persists with this or any exercise then you should stop until you talk to your physician or physical therapist.
2. Bend the left side of the head toward the left shoulder. If you feel pain or resistance, do not force the motion.
3. Bend the head back as far as possible without forcing any movement. If you feel pain or dizziness, stop until you talk to your physician or physical therapist.

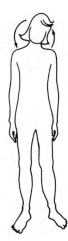

Figure 9. Diagram of neck exercise.

4. Bend the right side of the head to the right shoulder.
5. Turn to look over your right shoulder. Go as far as is comfortable, but do not force the movement.
6. Turn to look over your left shoulder. Go as far as is comfortable.

When you can do each of these exercises easily, repeat each exercise 2 times. Then you can gradually increase the repetitions to a total of 5 of each exercise, then 10 of each, then 20 of each. You may repeat this two or three times each day.

Shoulder Rotation

These exercises will increase the flexibility of the shoulders and arms. Increasing the number of repetitions also increases the strength of the arms. These exercises increase shoulder external rotation, the motion you use to comb your hair. You may sit, stand, or lie down to do this exercise (see Figure 10).

1. Clasp your hands behind your head. Pull your elbows together until they are as close as possible in front of your chin. Separate the elbows out to the side as much as possible.
2. Repeat this, gradually increasing to 5, then 10, then up to 20 repetitions. You may repeat these two or three times daily.

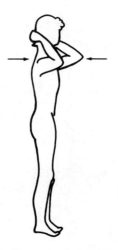

Figure 10. Diagram of shoulder rotation.

These exercises increase the flexibility of the shoulders and shoulder internal rotation, the motion women use to fasten a bra in the back or men use to put a wallet in a back pocket. This exercise is best done standing and is often done in the shower using a wash cloth to wash your upper back and a towel to dry your upper back (see Figure 11).

Shoulder flexion is the exercise you do when you raise your arms straight overhead (see Figure 12).

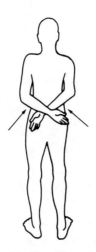 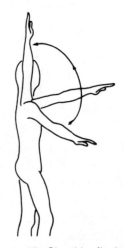

Figure 11. Shoulder rotation.   **Figure 12.** Shoulder flexion.

Shoulder abduction is the raising of the arms straight out to the side. If your arms hurt or you have difficulty raising them straight over your head when in a sitting or standing position, try lying on your bed and holding a stick (a broom handle will do).

1. Now raise your arms, keeping them straight and holding the stick with both hands, up over your head as far as possible. The less painful arm will help the painful arm go further.

2. Repeat this exercise, gradually increasing to 5, then 10, then 20 repetitions two or three times a day.

3. Now raise your arms out to the side, one at a time, and slowly make big circles (see Figure 13).

4. Repeat this exercise, gradually increasing to 5, then 10, then 20 repetitions two or three times a day.

This exercise can be done in a sitting or standing position and is fun to do during the day to relieve neck and shoulder tension and maintain shoulder girdle flexibility (see Figure 14).

1. Roll shoulders in a forward circle, raise shoulders towards ears in a shrugging motion, roll shoulders back and chest out as in a military stance, lower shoulders, and bring shoulders forward. Think of it as a simple shoulder roll in

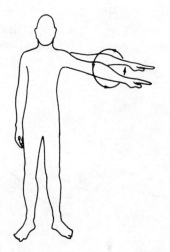

Figure 13. Shoulder abduction.

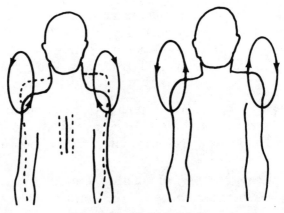

Figure 14. Shoulder girdle.

a circle. Now reverse the process, rolling your shoulder girdle in a backward circle.

2. Repeat this exercise, gradually increasing to 5, then 10, then 20 repetitions two or three times a day, if possible.

Hip Abduction

This exercise to improve the mobility of the hips is done lying on your bed or on the floor, whichever is the most comfortable for you (see Figure 15).

1. Lie on your back. Slide your legs as far apart as possible, one leg at a time, keeping your knee pointed to the ceiling.
2. Repeat this exercise increasing gradually to 5, then 10, then 20 repetitions two or three times a day, if possible.

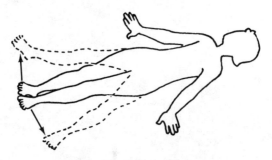

Figure 15. Hip abduction.

Hip Extension

The position for this exercise is lying on your stomach with one knee bent. This can be done on the bed or floor if you are able (see Figure 16).

1. Lift the thigh slightly off the floor or bed. If you lift too far you will rotate your pelvis and not get the desired movement. Now lift the other thigh. When you lift your thigh slightly off the floor try counting six seconds while you hold the motion. This is an isometric strengthening exercise to help build muscle strength. You may experience some cramping when you do this because your muscles are working hard to accomplish this motion. Try massaging the cramping muscle. If it persists, talk to your doctor or physical therapist.

2. Repeat this motion and gradually increase up to 5, then 10 repetitions if you can. Repeat this two times daily, if possible.

Hip Rotation

To do this exercise, lie on your bed or on the floor. This exercise may seem like a foot exercise but it actually rotates your hips when you keep your legs straight (see Figure 17).

1. Turn your knees in and touch your toes together. Now turn your knees and toes out.

2. Repeat this exercise, gradually increasing up to 5, then 10, then 20 repetitions each session. Repeat this exercise two times daily.

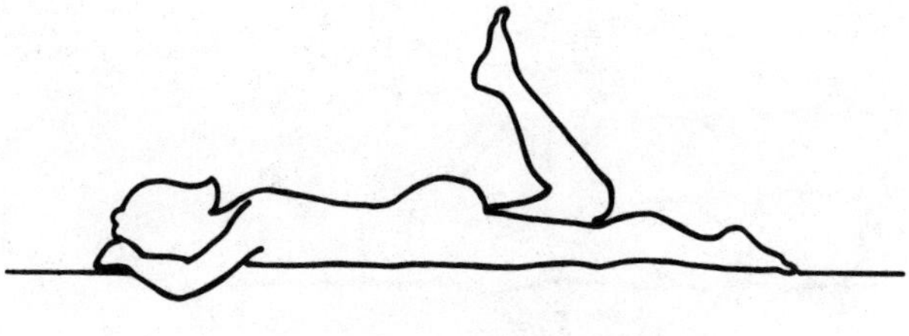

Figure 16. Hip extension.

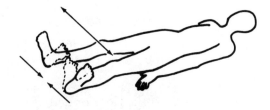

Figure 17. Hip rotation.

Hip Flexion and Back Stretching

This is a good exercise to do before you get out of bed in the morning to help you limber up for the day. It stretches the hips, the lower back, and knees. These exercises can be done on the bed or on the floor if you are able (see Figure 18).

1. Pull one knee at a time to your chest using your hands placed under your knee to help pull the leg further. Now do the same with the other leg. Repeat this alternating legs. Do 5, then 10, then 20 repetitions two or three times a day if possible.

2. Now pull both knees to your chest at the same time and hold for six seconds. Gently rock side to side while holding knees.

3. Repeat this exercise, increasing gradually to 5, then 10, then 20 repetitions two or three sessions a day if possible.

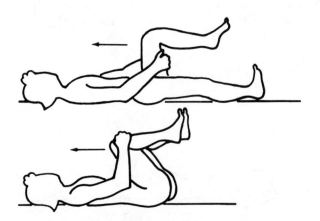

Figure 18. Hip flexion and back stretching.

Cheek to Cheek

This is a fun exercise because you can do it anywhere, any-time, and practically in any position. This exercise strengthens the muscles of the buttocks which help support the back and legs. When sitting, you will actually raise up out of the chair because of the contraction of the muscle group in the buttocks (see Figure 19).

1. Press your buttocks together and hold for a six-second count. Relax and repeat. Gradually increase up to 5, then 10, then 20 repetitions. Repeat two times daily.
2. This exercise can be done frequently during the day as tolerated wherever you may be.

Pelvic Tilt

This is one of the best exercises you can do to strengthen your abdominal muscles which in turn help support your back. This exercise will also help tone your stomach muscles. Do this exercise lying in bed or on the floor, whichever is more comfortable (see Figure 20).

1. Relax and raise your arms above your head. Keep your knees bent. Now comes the tricky part! Tighten the muscles of your lower abdomen and your buttocks as the same time to flatten your back against the bed or floor. This is the flat back position which you hold for a six second count. Now relax and repeat.

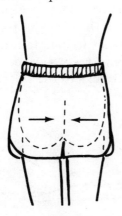

Figure 19. Cheek to cheek.

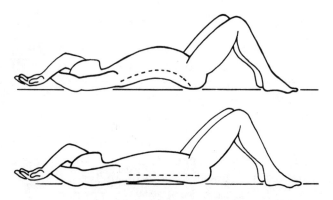

Figure 20. Pelvic tilt.

2. This is sometimes a difficult exercise to understand. If you have difficulty, contact your doctor or physical therapist and have them demonstrate the exercise.
3. Repeat this exercise 2 or 3 times to start and work gradually to 5, then 10, then 20 repetitions.
4. This exercise can also be done standing up or sitting in a chair but probably requires some demonstration by a therapist for these positions.

Bridging

This exercise is done lying in bed or on the floor. It strengthens the muscles in the back (see Figure 21).

1. Lie on the floor and bend (flex) your hips and knees. Now lift your hips and buttocks off the bed or mat 4 to 6 inches, forcing the small of the back out flat; and tighten the buttock and hip muscles to maintain this position. Hold this position for a count of six seconds. Now, relax and lower your hips and buttocks to the floor. Repeat.

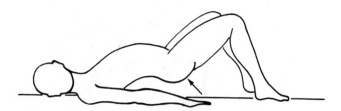

Figure 21. Bridging.

2. Repeat this exercise, gradually increasing up to 5, then 10, then 20 repetitions as tolerated. Repeat this twice daily if possible.

Straight Leg Raises

This exercise strengthens the muscles of the abdomen and improves the flexibility of the legs. Lie on your bed or on the floor, whichever is more comfortable for you (see Figure 22).

1. To protect your back during this exercise you will hug one leg to your chest, or simply bend the knee and hip, and rest the foot on the bed. See the picture for both positions. Choose the position most comfortable for you. Now raise the other leg straight up slowly as far as you can, trying to keep the abdomen in and maintaining the back firmly against the floor or bed as in the pelvic tilt-flat back position. When your back begins to arch, stop the raised leg at that point. Hold the position for six seconds. Bend and lower the leg, and repeat the exercise. Now do the same with the other leg.

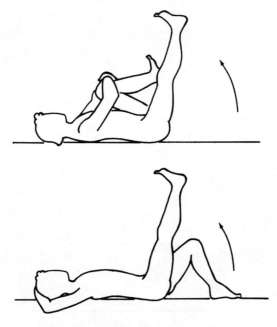

Figure 22. Straight leg raise.

2. Repeat this exercise, gradually increasing up to 5, then 10, then up to 20 repetitions. If your back hurts or you have pain in your leg, talk to your doctor or therapist before you continue.

Partial Sit Up

This is one of the more vigorous exercises you will do. It is an exercise to build abdominal strength which, in turn, better supports your back (see Figure 23).

To do this exercise lie on your bed or on the floor, whichever is the most comfortable for you.

1. Lie on your back with your knees bent. The goal of this exercise is to raise your head and shoulder blades off the floor. Now hold that position for a six-second count. Slowly return to the beginning position of lying on your back with your knees bent. Repeat.

2. Start this exercise slowly with 1 or 2 repetitions until your body adjusts to the exercise. Gradually increase to 5, then 10 repetitions. Be sure to do all strengthening exercises and count six seconds out loud as it is very important that you breathe properly while holding the position. By counting out loud you will surely breathe properly. If you experience shortness of breath, stop and talk to your doctor or physical therapist.

Back Extension

This exercise for strengthening the back muscles is done lying on your bed or the floor in a prone (stomach down) position (see Figure 24).

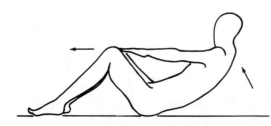

Figure 23. Partial situp.

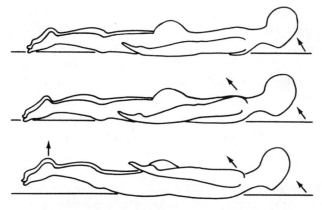

Figure 24. Back extension.

1. Raise your head, arms, and legs off the floor. Do not bend your knees. This must be done with your body straight in extension. Hold for several seconds while you count out loud. Relax and repeat.
2. Gradually increase this exercise up to 5, then 10 repetitions. If you experience discomfort, check with your doctor or physical therapist before you continue.

Cat Camel

Do not do this exercise for strengthening the back muscles if you have painful knees, ankles, or hands. It places pressure on these areas (see Figure 25).

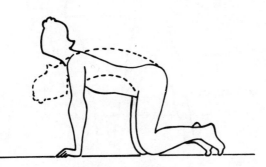

Figure 25. Cat camel.

1. The position for this exercise is a crawling position. Hands must be directly under your shoulders. Take a deep breath and arch your back as a frightened cat does, lowering your head. Hold that position while you count the six seconds out loud. Now exhale and drop the arched back slowly, raising your head.
2. Start this exercise slowly with 1 or 2 repetitions. Increase up to 5 and then 10 repetitions if possible.

Wall Push

This exercise is especially good for osteoporosis patients because it encourages the body extension positions (see Figure 26).

1. Stand spread eagle against a solid wall. Now arch your back inwards slowly.
2. Repeat this exercise and gradually increase repetitions from 1 to 5 or more. This exercise is fun because you can do it any time you feel you need a good body stretch. Repeat two times daily.

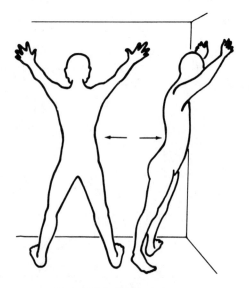

Figure 26. Wall push.

Deep Breathing

This exercise improves the movement of the chest and helps your posture. This exercise is performed in the rest position with your hands comfortably placed behind your head. You will also do a good shoulder rotation exercise by placing your hands behind your head. This position allows your rib cage and chest to expand fully. Bend your knees to protect your back (see Figure 27).

1. Once you are in this comfortable position, breathe deeply and raise your chest while filling your lungs completely. Hold for about two seconds and then exhale by drawing your upper abdomen in. Take the next breath against the uplifted chest. This may be a difficult exercise to understand without a demonstration. Contact your physical therapist or physician for assistance.
2. Begin this exercise slowly and gradually increase the repetitions from 5 to 10, then up to 20.

Wing Back

This is another exercise that is especially good for patients with osteoporosis because it encourages the bending of the arms and body backwards (see Figure 28).

1. This exercise is done in a relaxed standing position. Lift your elbows to shoulder height with arms bent. Now straighten arms backwards. Hold.
2. Repeat this exercise and gradually increase repetitions. Start with 5 and work up to 10, then 20 as tolerated. Repeat the exercise two times daily.

Arm Swing

The object of these exercises is to emphasize extension of the back and neck and increased expansion of the chest. All

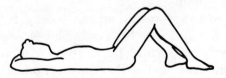

Figure 27. Deep breathing.

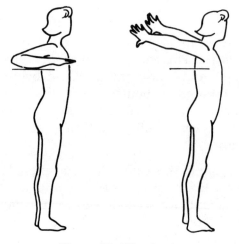

Figure 28. Wing back.

of these motions are important for patients with osteoporosis. Posture is important when doing these exercises. Stand comfortably with your knees, back, and shoulders slightly relaxed (see Figure 29).

1. Start with your hands down and crossed in front of you. Swing them slowly up and out over the head, reaching back as far as you can. When your arms are up take a deep breath. When you lower your arms exhale. Repeat.

2. Repeat this exercise, gradually increasing up to 5, then 10 repetitions. This exercise should be repeated two times daily.

Knee Extension

Sit in a chair and support your foot on a table or chair that is of comfortable height. This is a two-fold exercise (see Figure 30).

1. By simply straightening your leg you are maintaining knee flexibility. Make it as straight as you can tolerate and hold at that point.

2. Now, to add an isometric strengthening exercise, try pulling your toe up so the back of the leg is stretched. Tighten the knee cap by pushing the knee down a little bit and hold the contraction. You will notice wrinkles in the kneecap and the muscles in the thigh tighten. Hold that contraction

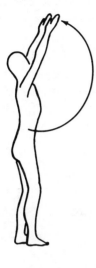
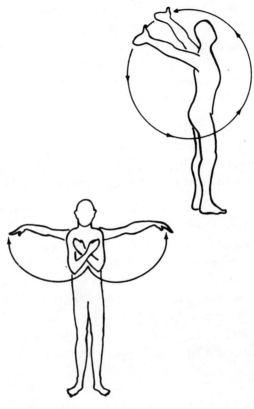

Figure 29. Arm swing.

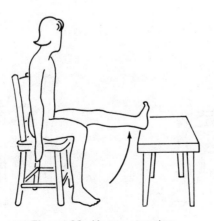

Figure 30. Knee extension.

for six seconds, relax, and repeat. This exercise is especially important for knee stability and standing support.

3. This is a very important exercise to maintain knee strength. Begin gradually and work up to 12 repetitions at one time. Repeat this two to three times a day. This exercise can be done while you relax in a chair watching television, or at work for a change of position and release of tension.

Ankles and Feet

This exercise increases flexibility and strength in the ankles and feet. The best position for this exercise is sitting in a chair with your feet flat on the floor (see Figure 31).

1. Now raise your toes as high as you can while keeping your heels down (see Figure 32).
2. Keep your toes down and lift your heels as high as possible.
3. Lift the inside of each foot and roll the weight over on the outside of the foot. Keep your toes curled down, if possible. The soles of your feet should be turned in facing each other (see Figure 33).
4. Rotate the ankle in a circle curling toes up and down and around in a circle (see Figure 34).

Wrist and Hand

To maintain mobility or flexibility in the wrist, use the other hand to bend the wrist as far as possible. Support your

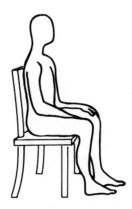

Figure 31. Ankle and foot.

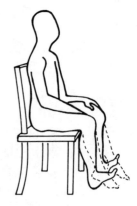

Figure 32. Ankle and foot.

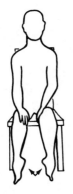
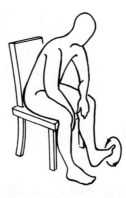

Figure 33. Ankle and foot.   **Figure 34.** Ankle and foot.

arm on a table or on the arm of a chair. Avoid holding the arm in mid-air when doing these exercises (see Figure 35).

1. Place the hand over the edge of a table and use the other hand to bend the hand up as far as possible. Now use the other hand to bend the hand down as far as possible.
2. Go as far as you can bend the hand easily. Repeat this, gradually increasing up to 5, 10, then 20 repetitions each session. Repeat the session two times daily.

This is a simple exercise which accomplishes the very important function of prehension and pinch in your finger and hand (see Figure 36).

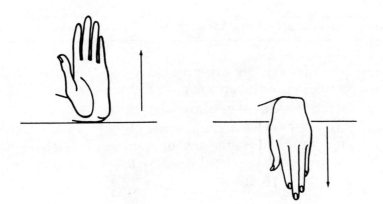

Figure 35. Wrist mobility.

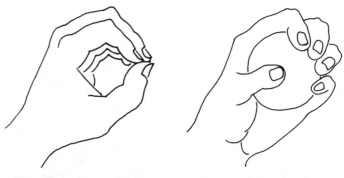

Figure 36. Making O's.   **Figure 37.** Squeeze ball.

1. Try to form the letter "O" with the thumb and each finger on the hand. After you make the "O," straighten the fingers and touch the next finger. Make an "O" and then straighten. Be sure the thumb rounds into a good "O."
2. Repeat this gradually increasing up to 5, then 10 repetitions. Repeat this exercise two times daily.

Use a *foam* rubber ball, slightly larger than a tennis size ball, and squeeze and release for this exercise. Make sure all your fingers close as far as possible around the ball. Release and straighten the fingers. It is important that you use a foam ball rather than a rubber ball. Foam balls are available at toy stores (see Figure 37).

════════ SUMMARY ════════

1. A regular exercise program is an important part of the prevention and treatment of osteoporosis.
2. Exercises are most effective when done properly.
3. Start exercises slowly and gradually after instruction by your physical therapist or your physician. If you have pain or discomfort, stop until you have talked to your physical therapist or physician.

CHAPTER EIGHT

A Calcium Guide for Strong Bones

Although calcium alone may not halt the progression of osteoporosis, research does indicate that increasing the amount of calcium in the diet may slow the development of the disease. When combined with other preventive measures and methods of treatment such as weight-bearing exercise, vitamin D, and medications, it is likely that calcium is effective in building bone density, especially when prevention is started in childhood years.

The Recommended Daily Allowance for calcium for an adult is 1000 mg per day. Experts on osteoporosis think that pre-menopausal women need 1000 mg per day and post-menopausal women need 1500 mg per day to prevent osteoporosis.

Calcium supplements can be used to ensure the proper amounts of calcium in the diet, but you need to check to figure the exact amount of calcium actually consumed. For example, although calcium carbonate generic tablets contain 500 mg of calcium carbonate, only 200 mg is actually taken in by the body. (See Calcium Supplement Chart, Table 11.)

Dietary calcium can be increased easily by including three or four servings of calcium-rich foods each day. We have listed many excellent sources of calcium that are available. This calcium guide should assist you and your family in meal planning that guarantees adequate calcium in the daily diet. Be sure to

TABLE 11
Some Calcium Supplements

Name	Type of Calcium	Actual Amount of Calcium
Posture	calcium	1200 mg/tablet
Tums tablets	calcium carbonate 500 mg tablet	200 mg/tablet
Tums E-X tablets	calcium carbonate 750 mg tablet	300 mg/tablet
Digel tablets	calcium carbonate 280 mg tablet	112 mg/tablet
Alkamints tablets	calcium carbonate 850 mg tablet	340 mg/tablet
Biocal calcium supplement tablets	calcium carbonate 1250 mg tablet	500 mg/tablet
Biocal calcium supplement chewables	calcium carbonate 625 mg/tablet	250 mg/tablet
Calcium carbonate tablets, generic	calcium carbonate 500 mg/tablet	200 mg/tablet
Calcium carbonate oral suspension	calcium carbonate 1250 mg/tsp.	500 mg/tsp.
Cal-Sup tablets	calcium carbonate 750 mg/tablet	300 mg/tablet
Dorcal children's liquid supplement	glubionate calcium 1800 mg/tsp.	115 mg/tsp.
Neo-Glucagon syrup	glubionate calcium 1800 mg/tsp	115 mg/tsp.
Os-Cal 500 tablets	oyster shell, 1250 mg	500 mg/tablet
Calcium gluconate tablets, generic	calcium gluconate 500 mg	45 mg/tablet
Calcium lactate tablets, generic	calcium lactate 650 mg	84.5 mg/tablet
Titralac tablets	calcium carbonate 420 mg/tablet	168 mg/tablet

use the following calcium guide and the fast food and convenience food guide to plan your meals.

Ways to Increase Calcium in Your Diet

- Include 3 to 4 servings of calcium-rich products daily in your diet. Milk, cheese, and yogurt all contain lactose which enhances calcium absorption.
- If you are counting calories, do not exclude the dairy products, but select low-fat or skim milk products.
- Vitamin D also enhances intestinal absorption of calcium. Therefore, sun exposure, which allows the body to make vitamin D, and drinking vitamin D-fortified milk can be helpful.
- Avoid a diet high in fat and protein, as excessive fat and protein can interfere with calcium absorption in the intestine.
- Avoid excessive intake of soft drinks and convenience foods containing food additives. High levels of phosphorus and phosphates can result in calcium loss from the bones.
- Other sources of calcium include salmon with bones, sardines, and green leafy vegetables. However, the oxalate content of green leafy vegetables like spinach and broccoli may decrease the absorption of calcium.
- Caffeine in coffee has also been implicated in calcium loss, so avoid excessive intake.

A Calcium Guide for Strong Bones

Table 12, a list of the calcium content of some common foods, is meant to help you guide your choices of foods. The values given for calcium in these foods are averages and are not meant to be exact. Foods vary in calcium content with ingredients and preparation. Try to use these values to understand which foods and which groups of foods are high in calcium. Milk and cheese products commonly contain higher amounts of calcium. Many food products have the calcium content on the package label.

TABLE 12
Calcium Content in Milligram of Selected Foods

Food	Portion	Calcium Content
Beverages		
Alcoholic		
Beer	12 oz.	20
Eggnog	4 oz.	45
Gin	1 oz.	0
Wine	4 oz.	5–10
Coffee, brewed	12 oz.	trace
Carbonated drinks		
Cola type drinks	12 oz.	0–trace
Ginger ale	12 oz.	trace
Mineral water	8 oz.	33 (varies)
Orange soda	12 oz.	trace
Root beer	12 oz.	trace
Noncola type drink	12 oz.	trace
Noncarbonated drinks		
Apple juice	6 oz.	10
Cranberry juice	6 oz.	10
Fruit punch	6 oz.	12
Punch	8 oz.	20
Orange juice with added calcium	6 oz.	200–300
Tea	8 oz.	trace
Water, drinking	8 oz.	varies
Bread, Grain, Cereal, Pasta Products		
Bagel	1 medium	20
Biscuit, 2″ diameter, average	1	40
Bread, sliced, cracked wheat	1 slice	20
Raisin bread	1 slice	25
Rye	1 slice	25
White, enriched	1 slice	25
Whole wheat	1 slice	25
Cornbread, whole ground meal	1 piece	95
Corn grits, enriched, cooked	1 cup	2
Dry cereal made with ½ cup milk	1 oz.	150–350
Farina made with milk	¾ cup	150
Fettuccine, cheese sauce	2 oz.	40
Flour, self-rising	1 cup	300
Wheat, all purpose	1 cup	20
White, all purpose	1 cup	18–20

TABLE 12 *(continued)*

Food	Portion	Calcium Content
Lasagna, cheese	8 oz.	220
Macaroni, baked with cheese	1 cup	360
Canned with cheese	1 cup	199
Cooked	1 cup	15
Frozen, with cheese	1 cup	235
Manicotti, cheese-filled	8.5 oz.	300–550
Muffin, refined flour	1	35–90
Noodles	1 cup	15
Oat bran, made with milk	1 oz.	150
Oatmeal, made with milk	1 oz.	160–170
Pancakes, buckwheat, 4″ diameter	4	230–390
Made with enriched flour	4	150–190
Pizza, cheese, 10″ diameter, ¼″ thick	1 pizza	620
Rice, converted, before cooking	1 cup	59–65
Brown, before cooking	1 cup	60
White, before cooking	1 cup	45
White, cooked	1 cup	15–20
Roll, breakfast, danish	1 roll	20
Refined flour	1 roll	15–30
Whole wheat	1 roll	34–45
Spaghetti, enriched, cooked	1 cup	14
Tomato sauce, cheese	1 cup	80
Stuffing, bread	½ cup	35–45
Tortilla	1	45
Waffles, frozen	2 small	40–90
Made fresh	1 large	180
Chips and Snacks		
Cheese puffs	1 oz.	16
Cheese straws, 5″ long	10 pieces	150
Corn chips	1 oz.	30–40
Potato chips	10 chips	8
Pretzels	10	6
Tortilla chips	1 oz.	35
Tortilla chips, cheese flavored	1 oz.	50
Dairy Products		
Butter	1 Tbsp.	3
Buttermilk, cultured	8 oz.	300
1% lowfat	8 oz.	300

TABLE 12 (continued)

Food	Portion	Calcium Content
Cheese		
American cheese spread	1 oz.	175
Blue cheese	1 oz.	140
Camembert cheese	1 oz.	30
Cheddar cheese	1 oz.	210
Cheddar cheese, grated	1 cup	845
Colby cheese	1 oz.	200
Cottage cheese, 1% milkfat	8 oz.	140
2% milkfat	8 oz.	150
4% milkfat	8 oz.	214
Creamed	8 oz.	150
Cream cheese	1 oz.	18
Edam cheese	1 oz.	200
Feta cheese	1 oz.	135
Gouda cheese	1 oz.	190
Monterey cheese	1 oz.	200
Parmesan cheese, grated	1 Tbsp.	65
Hard	1 oz.	325
Reduced calorie, low fat cheese	1 oz.	200
Ricotta cheese	1 oz.	110
Roquefort cheese	1 oz.	175
Sliced cheese, American	1 oz.	150–200
Jalapeno	1 oz.	200
Monterey Jack	1 oz.	200
Souffle, cheese	1 cup	191
Swiss cheese	1 oz.	270–300
Chocolate drink	8 oz.	250
Chocolate milk, 1% lowfat	8 oz.	300
Cream, light	½ cup	130
heavy	½ cup	90
Evaporated milk, regular, skim	8 oz.	500–600
Evaporated condensed milk	8 oz.	800
Goat's milk	8 oz.	300
Ice cream, most flavors	1 cup	175–270
Ice cream stick, vanilla, average	1	60
Instant meal drink made with milk	8 oz.	400–500
Milk, cow's milk, calcium-fortified	8 oz.	500
High protein	8 oz.	350
Lactose-reduced	8 oz.	300
Skim	8 oz.	300

TABLE 12 *(continued)*

Food	Portion	Calcium Content
Milk *(cont.)*		
2%	8 oz.	300
Whole milk	8 oz.	300
Milkshake, average vanilla	8 oz.	450
Average chocolate	8 oz.	400
Shake mix, average	8 oz.	300
Mousse	½ cup	100
Non-fat dry milk, prepared	8 oz.	300
Puddings, canned, most flavors	5 oz.	100
Cooked, made with milk	½ cup	150–250
Instant	½ cup	150–250
Sugar-free instant	½ cup	150
Pudding on a stick	1	75
Sour cream	1 Tbsp.	14
Welsh Rarebit	1 cup	582
White Sauce, medium	1 cup	288
Yogurt, frozen, high calcium	8 oz.	300
Frozen, most flavors	6 oz.	150
Frozen yogurt stick	2 ½ oz.	100–150
Nonfat	8 oz.	450
1% milkfat	8 oz.	400
1.5% milkfat	8 oz.	350
Soft frozen yogurt	3 oz.	60
Desserts and Sweets		
Bread pudding	1 cup	280
Cakes, angel food	1 slice	2–40
Chocolate, chocolate icing	1 slice	70
Cupcake with icing	1	23–35
Fruitcake, average	1 slice	10–30
Gingerbread, average	1 piece	60–80
Pound cake	1 slice	6–15
Sponge cake	1 slice	10–25
White, chocolate icing	1 slice	60–90
Yellow, chocolate icing	1 slice	60–80
Candies, caramels	1 oz.	40
Chocolate chips	1 oz.	25
Fudge, plain	1 oz.	20–30
Hard candies	1 oz.	0
Marshmallow, large	1	1

TABLE 12 *(continued)*

Food	Portion	Calcium Content
Milk chocolate	1 oz.	65
Peanut brittle	1 oz.	10
Cookies, average size		
Animal cookies	10	14
Brownie	2 large	15
Chocolate	1	10
Chocolate chip	1	8
Fig bars	1	11
Gingersnaps	1	5
Graham crackers	1	6
Oatmeal	1	7–15
Peanut butter	1	5–12
Sugar	1	6
Custard, homemade with milk, eggs	½ cup	145
Coconut	½ cup	140
Doughnuts, cake type	1	6–25
Gelatin, made with water	1 cup	0
Honey	2 oz.	2–4
Ice cream—see *Dairy Products*		
Ices, flavored	1 cup	0
Jams, preserves	1 Tbsp.	4
Jellies	1 Tbsp.	1–4
Molasses, blackstrap	1 Tbsp.	135
Cane, refined	1 Tbsp.	30–60
Pie, ⅛ of 9″ diameter pie		
Apple	1 slice	10
Banana cream	1 slice	130
Butterscotch	1 slice	86
Cherry	1 slice	15–20
Custard	1 slice	70–150
Lemon meringue	1 slice	14–24
Mincemeat	1 slice	20–45
Pumpkin	1 slice	45–95
Puddings—see *Dairy Products*		
Sherbet	1 cup	95
Sugar, brown, dark	1 cup	165
Granulated	1 cup	0–trace
Syrup, maple	2 Tbsp.	40–60
Table blends	2 Tbsp.	18
Tapioca cream pudding	1 cup	170–250

TABLE 12 *(continued)*

Food	Portion	Calcium Content
Eggs		
Boiled egg	1 large	28
Egg substitute, average	4 oz.	25–75
Egg substitute with cheese	4 oz.	28–78
Fish and Seafoods		
Clams, steamed or canned	8 oz.	121
Cod, broiled	1 steak	64
Crabmeat, cooked	1 cup	65
Flounder, baked	1 oz.	7
Haddock, fried	3 oz.	11–40
Herring, kippered	1 small	13–45
Lobster, steamed	1 pound	300
Oysters, raw, 13–19 medium	1 cup	226
Salmon, canned	3 oz.	160–250
Red with bones	3.5 oz.	195–350
Sardines, canned with bones	8 medium	350–450
Scallops, breaded, fried	3.5 oz.	110
Shad, baked	1 oz.	7
Shrimp, steamed	3 oz.	95
Swordfish, broiled	1 steak	37
Tuna, canned	3 oz.	6
Clam chowder	1 cup	37–170
Fritters	1 fritter	30
Codfish cakes, fried	2 small	0
Crab, deviled (2″ diameter)	1 cup	113
Imperial	1 cup	132
Fish sticks	4	12
Lobster Newburg	1 cup	218
Salad	½ cup	94
Oyster stew, made with milk	1 cup	280
Tuna salad	1 cup	41
Fruit		
Apple juice, fresh or canned	1 cup	15
Apples, raw	1 large	10
Canned or stewed	1 cup	10
Apricots, canned in syrup	1 cup	30
Dried, uncooked	1 cup	90
Fresh	3 medium	20
Nectar, or juice	1 cup	20

TABLE 12 *(continued)*

Food	Portion	Calcium Content
Avocado	½ large	10
Banana	1 medium	10
Blackberries, fresh	1 cup	45
Blueberries, canned	1 cup	20
Fresh	1 cup	20
Frozen	1 cup	20
Cantaloupe	½ medium	40
Cherries, canned, pitted,		
Unsweetened	1 cup	40
Fresh, raw	1 cup	35
Dates, dried	1 cup	105
Figs		
Fresh, raw	3 medium	55
Stewed or canned with syrup	3 medium	10
Fruit cocktail, canned	1 cup	20
Grapefruit, canned sections	1 cup	30
Fresh, (5″ diameter)	½	15
Juice	1 cup	20
Grapes, concord	1 cup	15
Muscat	1 cup	20
Grape juice, bottled	1 cup	30
Lemon juice	½ cup	10
Lemonade, frozen (concentrate)	6 oz.	10
Limeade, frozen (concentrate)	6 oz.	20
Olives, canned, large, green	10	25
Canned, large, ripe	10	60
Oranges, fresh, large	1	55–80
Orange juice, with added calcium	6 oz.	200–300
Papaya, fresh, cubed	1 cup	30
Peaches, canned, sliced	1 cup	10
Fresh	1 medium	14
Pears, canned, sweetened	1 cup	15
Raw, 2½″ × 3″	1 medium	20
Persimmons, Japanese	1 medium	10
Pineapple, canned, sliced	1 cup	30
Crushed	1 cup	30
Raw, diced	1 cup	25
Plums, canned in syrup	1 cup	25
Raw, 2″ diameter	1	10
Prunes, cooked (unsweetened)	1 cup	50
Prune juice (unsweetened)	1 cup	35

TABLE 12 *(continued)*

Food	Portion	Calcium Content
Raisins, dried	½ cup	50
Raspberries, frozen	½ cup	15
Rhubarb, cooked (sweetened)	1 cup	120
Strawberries, frozen	1 cup	35
Raw	1 cup	35
Tangerines, fresh	1 medium	35
Watermelon, 4" × 8"	1 wedge	30
Meat and Poultry		
Bacon, cooked crisp and drained	2	2
Beef, corned beef	3 oz.	20
Chuck, pot roast	3 oz.	9
Dried, chipped beef	3 oz.	15
Ground lean	3 oz.	11
Hamburger, commercial	3 oz.	10
Roast beef (oven-cooked)	3 oz.	10
Steak, round	3 oz.	13
Steak, sirloin	3 oz.	10
Chicken, broiled	3 oz.	7
Fried, breast, leg or thigh	3 oz.	7
Roasted	3 oz.	7
Duck	3 oz.	9
Lamb, chop, broiled	4 oz.	11
Pork, chop, thick	3 oz.	8
Ham, canned	2 oz.	5
Turkey, roasted	3 oz.	9
Veal, cutlet, broiled	3 oz.	9
Beef, cooked	1 slice	12
Beef and cheese enchiladas	8 oz.	310
Chili con carne with beans	1 cup	82
Chili con carne without beans	1 cup	14
Pot pie (4½" diameter)	1 pie	35
Ravioli, with beef	7½ oz.	34
Spaghetti, meatballs, cheese	1 cup	125
Stew, vegetables	1 cup	30
Brains, beef, calf, pork, sheep	3½ oz.	10
Chicken, a la king	1 cup	127
Chow mein	1 cup	58
Devine, prepared with milk	7 oz.	174
Fricassee, prepared	1 cup	14

TABLE 12 *(continued)*

Food	Portion	Calcium Content
Chicken (*cont.*)		
Pot pie (4½″ diameter)	1 pie	40
Frankfurter, beef, 7″ long	2	12
Heart, beef, sauteed with oil	3 oz.	6
Calf, 1 large slice	3 oz.	3
Chicken	3 medium	3
Lamb, 2 slices	3 oz.	12
Pork, 2 slices	3 oz.	3
Liverwurst	2 oz.	4
Luncheon meats, Bologna, (4″ diameter)	2 slices	7
Dried chipped beef	3 oz.	15
Ham	2 oz.	5
Roast beef	1 slice	12
Pork, ham, canned, spiced	2 oz.	5
Ham, croquette	1	45
Ham, luncheon meat	2 oz.	5
Pork, bacon, cooked and drained	2	2
Sausage, bulk	3½ oz.	7
Sweetbreads, calf, braised	3½ oz.	7
Tongue, beef	3 oz.	7
Nuts		
Almonds, dried	½ cup	170
Roasted and salted	½ cup	185
Brazil nuts	½ cup	130
Cashews	½ cup	30
Coconut, shredded	½ cup	10
Peanut butter (commercial)	⅓ cup	50
Peanuts, roasted	⅓ cup	40
Pecans, raw	½ cup	35
Sesame seeds, dry	½ cup	85
Sunflower seeds	½ cup	90
Walnuts, raw	½ cup	60
Oils, Fats, and Shortening		
Butter	1 Tbsp.	35
Hydrogenated cooking fat	1 cup	0
Lard	1 cup	0
Margarine	1 Tbsp.	5
Margarine	½ cup	20

TABLE 12 *(continued)*

Food	Portion	Calcium Content
Mayonnaise	1 Tbsp.	5
Oils		
Corn, safflower, soy bean oils	1 Tbsp.	0
Olive oil	1 Tbsp.	0
Peanut oil	1 Tbsp.	0
Salad dressing		
Blue and Roquefort cheese	2 Tbsp.	25
French	2 Tbsp.	5
Italian	2 Tbsp.	5
Russian	2 Tbsp.	5
Thousand Island	2 Tbsp.	5
Soups, Canned and Prepared		
Asparagus (prepared with milk)	8 oz.	175
Bean with pork, (prepared with milk)	8 oz.	285
Beef noodle	8 oz.	15
Beef vegetable	8 oz.	15
Broccoli, (prepared with milk)	8 oz.	285
Cheese, (prepared with milk)	8 oz.	275
Chicken or Turkey, (without milk)	8 oz.	25
Chicken gumbo	8 oz.	40
Chicken noodle	8 oz.	10
Chicken with rice	8 oz.	5
Chicken vegetable	8 oz.	15
Clam chowder, Manhattan type	8 oz.	75
Clam chowder, New England type	8 oz.	190
Cream soups, chicken, turkey, celery, mushroom, potato	8 oz.	100–215
Minestrone	8 oz.	35
Split-pea, with milk	8 oz.	180
Split-pea, with water	8 oz.	30
Tomato, with milk	8 oz.	170
Tomato, with water	8 oz.	15
Vegetable beef	8 oz.	10
Vegetable, vegetarian	8 oz.	20
Vegetables		
Artichoke, globe	1 large	60
Asparagus, green	6 spears	20

TABLE 12 *(continued)*

Food	Portion	Calcium Content
Beans, baked beans	1 cup	150
Black beans	1 cup	270
Garbanzo beans, canned	1 cup	150
Green beans, snap	1 cup	80
Lima, cooked	1 cup	80
Navy, baked with port	1 cup	95
Red kidney beans, canned	1 cup	75
Bean sprouts, uncooked	1 cup	20
Beets, cooked	1 cup	25
Beets, greens, steamed	1 cup	145
Broccoli, steamed	1 cup	135
Brussels sprouts, steamed	1 cup	50
Cabbage, as coleslaw (with Mayonnaise)	1 cup	50
Sauerkraut, canned	1 cup	85
Steamed cabbage	1 cup	65
Carrots, cooked, diced	1 cup	50
Raw, grated	1 cup	40
Strips, from raw	2 oz.	20
Cauliflower, steamed	1 cup	25
Celery, cooked, diced	1 cup	50
Stalk, raw	1 cup	45
Chard, steamed, leaves	1 cup	130
Collards, steamed	1 cup	35
Corn, steamed	1 ear	5
Canned	1 cup	10
Fritters	1	22
Cucumbers, 1/8" slices	1 cup	5
Dandelion greens, steamed	1 cup	300
Eggplant, steamed	1 cup	25
Endive	1 cup	45
Kale, steamed	1 cup	205
Lentils	1 cup	50
Lettuce, green, iceberg	1/4 head	20
Mushrooms, raw	1 cup	10
Mustard greens, steamed	1 cup	200
Okra, steamed	1 cup	150
Onions, cooked	1 cup	50
Raw, green	1 cup	65
Parsnips, steamed	1 cup	70

TABLE 12 (continued)

Food	Portion	Calcium Content
Peas, green, canned	1 cup	50
Fresh, steamed	1 cup	35
Frozen	1 cup	30
Pickles, cucumber, dill, large	1 pickle	35
Potatoes, baked	1 medium	15
Chips	10	10
French fries	10	10
Mashed with milk and butter	1 cup	70
Potato salad	1 cup	80
Scalloped with cheese	1 cup	310
Steamed	1 medium	15
Sweet potato, baked with skin	1 potato	40
Sweet potato, canned	1 can	85
Rutabagas	½ cup	50
Soybeans	1 cup	130
Curd, (2½" × 2¾")	1 piece	155
Spinach, steamed	1 cup	170
Squash, summer	1 cup	45
Tomatoes, canned, whole	1 cup	55
Catsup	1 Tbsp.	5
Juice	1 cup	20
Raw	1 large	25
Turnip greens, steamed	1 cup	270
Watercress, raw, chopped finely	1 cup	190
McDonalds		
Egg McMuffin	1	226
Hotcakes with butter	1 serving	103
Scrambled eggs	1 serving	61
Pork sausage	1 serving	16
English muffin with butter	1	117
Hashbrown potatoes	1 serving	5.33
Biscuit with spread	1	74
Biscuit with sausage	1	82
Biscuit with sausage and egg	1	119
Sausage McMuffin	1	196
Apple Danish	1	14
Iced Cheese Danish	1	32.9
Cinnamon Raisin Danish	1	35
Raspberry Danish	1	14.2

TABLE 12 *(continued)*

Food	Portion	Calcium Content
Hamburger	1 (100 g)	84
Cheeseburger	1 (114 g)	169
Quarter pounder	1 (160 g)	98
Quarter pounder with cheese	1 (186 g)	255
Big Mac	1 (200 g)	203
Filet-O-Fish	1 (143 g)	133
McD. L. T.	1 (254 g)	250
Chicken McNuggets	109 g	11
French fries	1 serving	9
Apple pie	1 (85 g)	14
Vanilla milkshake	1 (291 g)	329
Chocolate milkshake	1 (291 g)	320
Strawberry milkshake	1 (290 g)	322
Soft serve ice cream and cone	1 (115 g)	183
Strawberry sundae	1 (164 g)	174
Hot fudge sundae	1 (165 g)	215
Hot caramel sundae	1 (165 g)	200
McDonaldland cookies	67 g	12
Chocolaty Chip cookies	69 g	29
Burger King		
Burger King Whopper Sandwich	1	84
Whopper with Cheese	1	215
Double Beef Whopper	1	95
Double Beef Whopper with Cheese	1	226
Whopper Jr. Sandwich	1	40
Whopper Jr. with Cheese	1	105
Bacon Double Cheeseburger	1	168
Hamburger	1	37
Cheeseburger	1	102
Whaler Sandwich	1	46
Ham and Cheese Sandwich	1	195
Chicken Sandwich	1	79
Salad, plain	1 serving	18
With House Dressing	1 serving	37
With Blue Cheese	1 serving	44
With Thousand Island	1 serving	66
With Reduced Calorie Italian	1 serving	42
Breakfast Croissan'wich	1	40
Bacon Egg, Cheese	1	136

TABLE 12 *(continued)*

Food	Portion	Calcium Content
Breakfast Croissan'wich *(cont.)*		
Sausage, Egg, Cheese	1	145
Ham, Egg, Cheese	1	136
Scrambled Egg Platter	1 serving	101
With sausage	1 serving	112
With bacon	1 serving	103
French Toast Sticks	1 serving	77
Great Danish	1	91
Onion Rings, regular	1 serving	124
Milk		
2% lowfat	1 cup	297
Whole	1 cup	290
Shakes, medium		
Vanilla	1	295
Chocolate	1	260
Vanilla (syrup added)	1	NA
Chocolate (syrup added)	1	248
Sandwiches		
Bacon, lettuce and tomato on white bread	1	53
Chicken salad on white bread	1	50
Corned beef on rye bread	1	50
Cream cheese and jelly on white bread	1	60
Egg salad on white bread	1	65
Ham on white bread	1	40
Hot dog on bun	1	65
Peanut butter and jelly on white bread	1	70
Roast beef on white bread	1	60
Tuna salad on white bread	1	48
Combination Foods		
Beans and franks	8 oz.	122
Beef pie	8 oz.	32
Beef vegetable stew	8 oz.	29
Beef stroganoff	6 oz.	24
Cabbage rolls	8 oz.	55
Cannelloni, beef, tomato sauce	8¼ oz.	298
Chicken, cheese sauce	8¼ oz.	389
Shrimp, cheese sauce	8¼ oz.	490

Winning with Osteoporosis

TABLE 12 *(continued)*

Food	Portion	Calcium Content
Chicken a la king	8 oz.	127
Chicken and noodles	8 oz.	26
Chicken and rice	8 oz.	122
Chicken parmigiana	7 oz.	174
Chicken pie	8 oz.	70
Chili con carne with beans	8 oz.	90
Without beans	8 oz.	80
Chicken chow mein	8 oz.	40–50
Enchiladas, beef and cheese	8 oz.	309
Enchiladas, cheese	12 oz.	425
Corn fritter	3½ oz.	64
Corned beef hash	10 oz.	65
Macaroni and cheese	12 oz.	220
Lasagna and cheese	8 oz.	220
Miscellaneous		
Featherweight baking powder	1 Tbsp.	1500

CHAPTER NINE

Case Studies: Patients Who Have Managed Their Osteoporosis

Do prevention and treatment work? In our clinic we see the results of treatment of osteoporosis daily. We regularly find that a person who is able to maintain a regular program, as outlined in Chapters Four and Five, improves. However, most people, even with advanced osteoporosis (Stages 3 and 4), may resume daily activity with minimal limitation. Each part of the program is important—exercise, medication, and risk factor removal. Those who don't improve usually cannot follow this regular program.

Let's look at specific examples of people who have managed their osteoporosis effectively. These are true cases from our clinic records with the names changed.

One case which we discussed in Chapter One is that of a 60-year-old woman who worked as a cashier. Nancy developed severe, constant back pain over 1 to 2 years from several compression fractures in the spine. She became more stooped and had constant severe pain. She was unable to continue her work. After the diagnosis of osteoporosis (Stage 4) was made, Nancy began a regular exercise program of back exercises and walking, began taking calcium, other medications, and quit smoking.

Over a period of months the pain decreased, her walking increased, and she returned to work as a cashier, a job that requires standing for several hours each day. She has had no further fractures.

Judy is a 55-year-old lady who was seen after one year of severe back pain which began while riding a horse. She was found to have osteoporosis and compression fractures in her spine. She began exercises and walking. She also began a treatment program involving calcium, other medications, and estrogen therapy. Over a period of about eight months her pain diminished to the point that it was no longer limiting. No further fractures have occurred. Bone density tests have shown improvement in osteoporosis after two years of treatment.

Barbara is a 60-year-old woman who has had severe rheumatoid arthritis for years. She developed several fractures of the spine requiring hospitalization. She was unable to tolerate medications including calcium, vitamin D, fluoride, and calcitonin. Her exercise and walking is limited by her severe arthritis. She has continued to have fractures and more limitation of activity, along with severe, constant back pain. Her limitations in following a treatment program have probably prevented improvement.

Elizabeth is a 19-year-old long distance runner. She developed a painful right foot while training, and had repeated fractures in the bones of the feet. All other tests were normal. Her intense level of training had caused her menstrual periods to stop. It is most likely that this resulted in loss of bone density and fracture. She lowered her level of training slightly, added estrogen treatment, and she has had no further fractures.

Mary is 65, lives in a retirement community, and suffered for three years with severe back pain. She became stooped and severely limited in activity. She was found to have advanced osteoporosis. She began a regular exercise and walking program, calcium, vitamin D, and calcitonin. She had nausea and was unable to tolerate fluoride treatment. After seven months she became able to walk 1 to 2 miles daily and is now known in her community as "the walker."

Another patient, June, is a 59-year-old woman who has smoked for 30 years. Her mother had severe osteoporosis with fractures in the hip and compression fractures in the spine. Her mother now walks very little due to severe pain in the back. Her father died after a fracture of a hip and prolonged illness in a nursing home. June has had no fractures but because of her risk factors had osteoporosis screening by bone density test. She was found to have significant osteoporosis. She has begun a program for treatment of Stage 2 osteoporosis. She has increased her calcium intake to 1500 mg daily, has begun a regular exercise and walking program, and has decreased cigarettes. She plans to stop smoking as soon as possible.

Only time will tell if June's efforts will strengthen her bones and avoid fractures. Knowing about risk factors allowed her to begin treatment at an earlier stage than would have been possible otherwise.

Susan is a 67-year-old woman who has had emphysema for many years. She saw a doctor one year ago because pain in the upper back limited her walking. She had been quite active, including playing golf, but was unable to continue because of the pain. She was diagnosed as having osteoporosis with fractures in the thoracic spine (the middle and upper part of the back). Her Stage 3 osteoporosis was treated with exercise for the back, walking, calcium, and other medications. After 9 or 10 months, Susan has resumed walking regularly and now plays golf again, although not yet at her previous level.

Osteoporosis is not just a woman's disease. Larry, a 65-year-old man, had pain in the lower back for years. He had learned to live with pain, and had retired from work as a welder. He smoked cigarettes for 20 years. He seldom ate dairy products. Several family members had suffered fractures, shortening of height, and stooped posture. He developed severe pain in the upper and middle parts of his back after lifting boxes during moving. Tests showed that he had osteoporosis with fractures in the spine. He was treated for this Stage 3 osteoporosis with exercises, walking, calcium, and other medications. He now is slightly stooped, but he had no pain in the upper back and has returned to his previous level of activity.

Fred, another 65-year-old man, is a retired executive. Fred was in excellent health and very active until he developed a medical problem which required prednisone, a cortisone-like medication, for treatment. This medical problem, temporal arteritis, was well-controlled with the medication. However, after a number of months of treatment, Fred developed severe pain in his right hip after a fall. He was found to have a fracture of the hip which has since been treated. Tests performed at that time showed that he had osteoporosis. It is possible that the prednisone, which was necessary to control his medical problem, contributed to the osteoporosis and fracture. This Stage 3 osteoporosis was treated. In addition, Fred continues to use the lowest possible dose of prednisone necessary to control his other problem.

Anyone can develop osteoporosis. With knowledge of the risk factors involved in osteoporosis, you can take action and begin prevention, management, and treatment of your specific stage.

Many examples of osteoporosis are available. We usually find improvement if a person is able to follow a regular program including:

• Removal of risk factors
• Regular exercise program
• Walking
• Proper medications

Improvement may not always occur in those people who cannot follow a regular program. These people may not be able to tolerate the medications, may be unable to follow a regular exercise program, or may be so discouraged that it is difficult to continue treatment.

It is unusual for a patient with osteoporosis not to improve if he or she follows these guidelines, even in far-advanced cases. It is never too early to begin prevention and never too late to consider proper treatment. Learn to managed osteoporosis, and you will be able to change the outcome of this disease.

Linda, a 58-year-old homemaker, thought that she was too young to have osteoporosis. Also, it did not run in her family. She recently had to care for her husband during a long illness which involved lifting and turning him frequently. Linda had a hysterectomy 10 years earlier at which time her ovaries were removed. She did not take estrogen treatments because of concern about possible side effects. She began to have severe pain in the middle part of her back. Linda was later found to have a compression fracture in the spine due to osteoporosis. No other underlying medical problems were found. She was treated with calcium and other medications. She now walks more than two miles daily and has occasional pain in the back, but is not limited in any activity.

Mary, a 70-year-old teacher developed severe back pain about six months after an operation for cancer of the intestine. Although the spread of cancer can cause back pain, she was found to have osteoporosis with a fracture of one of the vertebral bodies in the lower part of the back (lumbar spine). She improved after bedrest for one week and began a gentle exercise program under a therapist's supervision. Although she used a walker at first, she now walks unaided. Mary's Stage 3 osteoporosis is no longer severely limiting. Hopefully, her treatment will prevent future fractures, although there is no guarantee. It seems reasonable to continue this treatment.

Kay, an extremely active woman of 66, is a retired business executive. She developed pain in her left foot after walking on a vacation. Although she has arthritis in her feet, the pain seemed different to her. She had a small fracture in one of the bones in the foot. Bone density tests were performed that showed she had osteoporosis, but no other serious medical problems. The foot pain from the fracture has gradually decreased.

Who can get osteoporosis? As you can see by reading individual patient histories, anyone can. Osteoporosis is not just an older woman's disease. This disease can happen in men and women, young and old, although it is more common in the female sex. Prevention and immediate treatment are the keys to halting the devastating effects.

The more information you have on the prevention and treatment of osteoporosis—the better you can manage your osteoporosis.

SUMMARY

Preventing and treating osteoporosis is possible if a combination of exercise, medication, and removal of risk factors are included in the patient's daily lifestyle.

Osteoporosis can occur in men or women, young or old. It is never too early to begin prevention and never too late to consider proper treatment.

CHAPTER TEN

Questions
Patients Ask

We are confronted daily in our clinic with a multitude of questions concerning osteoporosis. These questions are from patients with osteoporosis, their family members, and persons who want to prevent the crippling disease.

Communication with your physician is vital in the treatment of any disease. We suggest that patients write down concerns they may have before the actual examination then ask the physician questions at the appropriate time.

By discussing your individual problem with your physician, you can learn specific ways to approach osteoporosis in a knowledgeable manner that will benefit you.

These are some of the questions we are asked most frequently.

Q: A young woman asks, "I am concerned about osteoporosis, especially after reading so many reports lately in magazines. My mother is in her mid-fifties and doesn't appear to have any risk factors other than being over the age of 40. Should she be taking action to prevent osteoporosis? Is there something we can do together?"

Most of us know a middle-aged or older woman who is at risk for osteoporosis. This may be a friend, a wife, an aunt, or a mother. Many of these women already have osteoporosis established and are at risk for a fracture. We must remember that osteoporosis may begin before age 40. These women have bones which have reached maturity and may be in the stage of gradual reduction in the total amount of bone density. They may have slightly more stooped posture than in earlier years. Their height may be slightly less than in their younger years.

As far as you and your mother are concerned, there are steps you both can take to delay or prevent further problems of osteoporosis such as fractures. Your mother might fit into Stage 1 or Stage 2 osteoporosis. In other words, the gradual loss of bone has begun but is not detectable (Stage 1) or enough loss of bone has occurred to be found by a bone density test (Stage 2) (Figure 38).

This is an excellent time for you both to begin prevention. This is the time when a little effort and trouble may allow a large savings later in illness, expense, and loss of activity.

If you or your mother have more than one or two risk factors, then the chances of osteoporosis are much increased. The

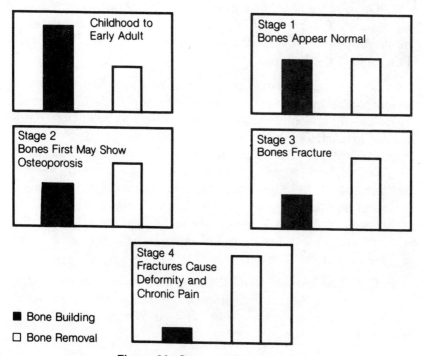

Figure 38. Stages of Osteoporosis.

more risk factors present, the greater the need for early action. This may be the only warning of osteoporosis before fractures in later years.

Your mother may want to discuss these risk factors and her situation with her physician. Depending on her set of risk factors and other health status, bone density tests will detect osteoporosis if it is present.

If more than one or two risk factors are present then your mother should consider specific prevention measures as outlined in Chapter Five. This may include calcium, exercise, and other measures. This action may delay or prevent further osteoporosis. If osteoporosis is found to be present by tests then there may be other measures taken, including the possibility of taking medicines. These treatments are outlined in Chapter Six.

It is best not to wait until a fracture draws attention to osteoporosis. The fracture may be very limiting (as examples in this book indicate), and will probably be expensive. It is never too early to start prevention of osteoporosis.

Q: A 68-year-old man asks, "Why do medications such as cortisone add to my risk of getting osteoporosis? I have had to take prednisone for years for asthma and wonder if it is too late to help my body. What should I do?"

You do have several risks. In most cases like yours, the likelihood of osteoporosis can be extremely high. Being 68-years-old, having lung disease for years, and requiring prednisone (a cortisone-like medication) all greatly increase your risk. Still, it is never too late to try to prevent future fractures. You should first try to remove all other risk factors if possible and pay attention to your calcium intake. If these measures are followed during the time of treatment of the lung disease with prednisone, you may be able to limit the negative effects of the drug. Bone density tests can tell if you have osteoporosis and whether other medications would be needed.

Q: A 63-year-old man asks, "My wife has been active most of her life until several months ago when she fractured her wrist while playing golf. Should she have further tests to determine if osteoporosis is present?"

This question raises a few important points. Wrist fractures are one of the most common types in osteoporosis (in addition to hip and spine fractures). Osteoporosis is the most likely problem in this sort of fracture, especially if it happened with only mild injury. If the bone strength had been normal, presumably a mild injury would not cause a fracture.

A few practical points are worthwhile to consider. Your orthopedic surgeon may be able to tell if the bones have osteoporosis from the wrist X-ray, although in many cases this is not possible. If the X-rays do not give an answer, ask your physician if an osteoporosis screening test or other tests should be done to confirm the osteoporosis. If no other medical problems are found then it may be useful to consider specific measures to try to prevent further fractures. Remember, if this is a fracture caused by weakness due to osteoporosis, it would suggest Stage 3, osteoporosis with fractures (Figure 39). The bones have gradually become less dense and have weakened enough that injuries which may have gone unnoticed earlier now result in fractures. Although this wrist fracture is the first symptom your wife exhibited, it has occurred quite a few years into the process of osteoporosis.

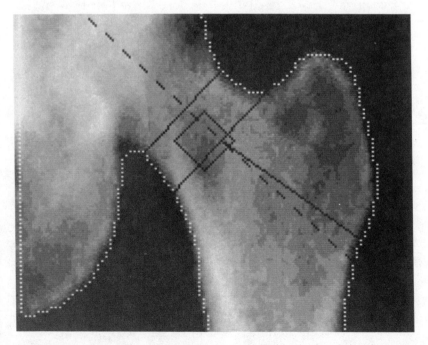

Figure 39. Areas of the hip and spine measured in the bone density test.

Treatment for Stage 3 is outlined in Chapter Six. This treatment includes removal of risk factors, addition of calcium to the diet, and perhaps other medications. This is an excellent time for your wife to begin managing her osteoporosis.

Q: A 47-year-old woman asks, "I had a hysterectomy several years ago. How do I know if my estrogen replacement is enough to halt osteoporosis?"

Because you had a hysterectomy at an earlier age than the average age of menopause, you may be at a higher risk for osteoporosis if the ovaries were also removed. A hysterectomy is frequently done for reasons which allow the surgeon to leave one or both ovaries in place. This allows the continued secretion of the female hormone estrogen until the time of menopause.

If the ovaries were also removed (oophorectomy) then estrogen therapy may be prescribed depending on your situation. Some women should not take estrogen therapy because of the possibility of side effects. Let your physician guide you in your own case. The dose of estrogen which most researchers feel is needed to prevent osteoporosis is usually the equivalent of 0.625 mg conjugated estrogen daily. This dose started near the time of menopause has been shown to slow the rate of bone loss and may actually increase the bone formation slightly. It is most effective when it is taken as soon as possible after menopause. The first few years after menopause seem to be the most critical in preventing the effects of the loss of estrogen levels in the body on the bone.

How long should estrogens be taken? The answer is not known. Research is now being done which may give an answer. Until then, most researchers feel that, if possible, estrogen therapy should continue for at least 10 to 15 years. At that time it may be stopped if desired. If there are side effects of the estrogen therapy then it may be stopped earlier. It should not be given if it causes serious problems.

If for some reason you are not able to take estrogen therapy after menopause, you should be more careful to remove other risk factors for osteoporosis. Through careful attention and proper action, you will be able to minimize your risk. If you are more than 15 years after menopause, let your physician help you decide if estrogen therapy is appropriate in your own situation.

Q: A mother of teenagers asks, "My daughters are constantly on the go. Although I try to prepare balanced diets with calcium-rich foods, they seem to leave a lot on their plates. How can I be sure that they will be protected in their growing years?"

What a common problem this is! Many families are so busy that they often don't eat together. As seen in Chapter Seven, calcium in the teenage years is important because it allows full development of the bone density at maturity. If the body does not have enough calcium during these rapidly growing years then it may not be able to give the maximum "supply" of bone to prepare for the possible loss of bone later in life. Research shows much of the body's bone growth happens during our teenage years. It is hard to predict which teenager will develop osteoporosis as an adult. Until we can better predict this, researchers tell us that it does seem to matter how well we build our bones during these rapid growth years. The person will not be able to feel any effect during the early years. But when the maximum supply of bone is built at an early age, that person will be more resistant to osteoporosis later in life.

Our busy schedules, combined with personal tastes in food, attempts to reduce calorie intake and control weight, make proper calcium intake difficult at times. Be as sure as possible of proper overall nutrition. Then if maintaining 1200 mg of calcium daily is still difficult, don't hesitate to add a calcium supplement for teenagers. Knowledge of calcium content of various foods, including fast foods, as shown in the tables in Chapter Six, will be useful. Also, education of teenagers can be effective. Help your teen find ways to be sure of calcium intake which can fit with her desires for weight control. We have found most teenagers are eager to learn and are capable of managing calcium in their diet.

Q: A 34-year-old woman asks, "I have been allergic to milk since infancy and have never supplemented with calcium tablets. But now I am concerned! Is it too late to help myself in avoiding osteoporosis?"

You have probably consciously avoided milk and dairy products throughout your life. Since these happen to be one of the main sources of calcium in our diet, it is probably safe to assume that you have a major risk factor of low calcium in the diet for many years. This makes you more likely to have developed bones that do not have the maximum density. Because you are probably close to your maturity as far as the bones are concerned, you may have to deal with a less-than-average amount of maximum bone. If you happen to develop osteoporosis later, you would have less total bone supply to last throughout your life. It is better to build the most possible bone density before maturity than to try to build more bone after we reach maturity.

You may have a true allergy to milk. If so, then you must avoid all milk products. It is common to have an intolerance to milk without a true allergy. This means a person may have abdominal pain, cramps, nausea, or diarrhea after drinking milk. There may not be a true allergic reaction. Intolerance may be caused by low or absent level of the enzyme lactase that is needed to digest milk. As a result, abdominal pain and diarrhea occur. Over the years, these persons usually learn not to consume milk products.

A product is now available that can be added to milk which corrects this lactase deficiency. It is sold at drug stores without a prescription and comes in drops or tablets which can be added to milk to prevent these problems. Also, some dairies add lactobacillus to milk which may help in some milder cases. Discuss this with your physician.

It is not too late for you to take proper action to help prevent osteoporosis in later years. You should simply supplement your diet with calcium as outlined in Chapter Five on page 63. You should remove any risk factors possible and consider taking estrogen replacements when you reach menopause (usually 45–55 years old). Avoidance of this risk factor may help protect you from future osteoporosis despite your lifelong low-calcium intake. Bone density testing may be helpful at some point to tell if osteoporosis is developing.

Q: A 29-year-old woman asks, "My grandmother recently had hip surgery after a fractured hip due to osteoporosis. She is 74 years old. How can I tell if I have osteoporosis now so I can avoid all the pain and suffering she has experienced recently?"

We feel the most important step is to be aware of the disease. You are at an ideal age for prevention of osteoporosis in later years. Your risk factors include female sex and a family history of osteoporosis. You should review the other major risk factors. If you have more than two then you should certainly begin specific preventative measures.

Despite your family history, bone density tests would tell if you have developed osteoporosis, but can't predict the future. This is because tests are not good enough to tell exactly how much bone formation and removal is happening at age 29. If the process leading to osteoporosis has begun, it is likely to be in Stage 1. The gradual change to less bone formation and more bone removal may have begun. The bones, however, are perfectly normal in strength at this point. But since you are at increased risk, it is important to take action now. If you wait until we can make the diagnosis of osteoporosis then you have lost the chance for prevention.

Prevention includes the measures outlined in Chapter Four, involving the removal of risk factors, a diet including an adequate calcium intake, and a good exercise program. Review the section in Chapter Four on prevention and discuss your situation with your physician to be sure you are doing all you can.

In later years (usually around age 40), it will be acceptable to have one of the osteoporosis screening tests done for your own piece of mind. This may also help guide any other treatment available at the time.

Q: An older man asks, "I have emphysema and have smoked most of my life although I recently stopped. I know that these are two of the risk factors for osteoporosis, but do men really have to worry about getting it as well?"

As we mentioned earlier, so much attention has been given to women that osteoporosis may be overlooked in men. Hip fractures are just as limiting, dangerous, and expensive in men as in women. By age 90, up to 17 percent of men may have hip fractures. If these and other fractures can be prevented it results in significant savings in suffering and expense. Risk factors which are common in men who develop osteoporosis are chronic lung disease such as emphysema and chronic bronchitis. Lung specialists commonly see men as well as women who have severe osteoporosis. It can be in part a result of the treatment of lung disease which, in some cases, requires cortisone-like medicines. These medicines increase the risk of osteoporosis but may be life-saving for these patients. The combination of cigarette smoking, emphysema, and cortisone-like medicines greatly increases the risk. Stopping cigarettes, treating the lung disease, and keeping the cortisone-like dose to a minimum can be helpful. Also, you can help by consuming proper amounts of calcium, exercising as allowed by your physician, and removing any other risk factors. Bone density tests can detect osteoporosis.

Q: A new mother asks, "Both my mother and grandmother have a 'dowager's hump,' and movement is painful. Having just delivered my first daughter, I am concerned about the chances I have of getting osteoporosis. How can I protect myself and my young daughter?"

"Dowager's hump" refers to the prominence in the upper part of the back that has the appearance of a hump. It is commonly seen in older women (dowagers). It is most commonly caused by a loss of height of the vertebral bodies, a symptom of osteoporosis. The shape changes and, as a result, so does the shape of the back. This change can happen with or without pain in the back, depending on the severity and other factors.

If the changes in your relatives' spines were from osteoporosis, you have a strongly positive family history. This is a risk factor that should not be ignored. It is no reason for alarm, but reason for enough concern to be careful to look for other risk factors. It should make the women in your family more aware of the disease and allow them the chance at an early age to prevent osteoporosis. It is not necessary to wait until it becomes obvious.

You can protect yourself by removing any other risk factors present, being sure of adequate calcium intake, maintaining a good exercise program, and other measures as outlined in Chapter Four.

Your daughter should have proper calcium intake as a young child. She should be taught proper diet and exercises as a child and teenager. If she is a finicky eater then she should be taught specific ways of ensuring enough calcium intake as suggested in Chapter Six. It is now thought that the larger the supply of bone mass that is built before we mature as an adult, the longer the bone will last if osteoporosis occurs.

Your mother and grandmother should also learn about osteoporosis. If present in these women, it is in an advanced stage and could suggest a higher risk of hip fracture. Hip fractures can be dangerous and limiting as you have seen. These usually require hospitalization, may require an operation, and greatly raise the cost of health care. A good place to start would be a review of the risk factors in Chapter Two. Then discuss bone density tests and treatment with your physician. At this stage, there are definite measures that can be taken to delay the progress of osteoporosis. Treatment does work.

Q: A 30-year-old woman asks, "You mention the lack of exercise as the first risk factor. Is this one the most important in determining the chances of osteoporosis occurring?"

It is not yet proven that exercise alone can prevent osteoporosis. In fact, we are still learning the role of exercise in this disease. But there is some interesting information available. Healthy people who have no exercise lose bone more rapidly. A good example of this is the bone loss that can happen to healthy astronauts on long, weightless space flights. Many researchers have shown that people who are bedridden may develop osteoporosis. And, in animals, activity and stress on bones seem to affect the way bones are produced. The strength of the bone is also affected. Some evidence supports that if our back muscles are made stronger, then the bone density and strength of the bones of the spine increases. Those people who exercise regularly over a long period of time seem to have fewer fractures.

Research is now under way in several centers to show how much and what kind of exercise is needed to prevent osteoporosis. Also, we need to know what sort of exercise program may help arrest osteoporosis once it has caused bone loss and fractures.

Until more is known, it seems reasonable to emphasize exercise for several reasons. Most patients who are able to begin and maintain a regular (even limited) exercise program seem to improve. The expense of such a program is low. You can do most of the exercises needed at home independently. If you have supervision and begin the program slowly and carefully, you can maintain a reasonable exercise program.

Q: A young woman asks, "My grandmother has moved in with our family. She still enjoys getting out for walks and going shopping. The problem is that she is embarrassed about her posture. Her stooped appearance seems to be making her depressed. How can I help her?"

It is reasonable to first confirm that your grandmother's stooped posture is caused by osteoporosis. Her physician will be able to tell whether other problems are present which need treatment. If osteoporosis is the main problem, then the stooped posture is probably a result of change in the shape of the vertebral bodies. (See the photograph shown in Figure 40 of the dowager's hump.) If several square vertebral bodies become compressed and wedge-shaped, the curve of the spine can change. If there is pain then the body tends to bend forward to decrease the pain. This adds to the stooped posture. The longer this posture is maintained, the more difficult it is to correct.

The stage of osteoporosis with deformity, Stage 4, can be difficult for the family and the patient as well. Often the pain has been considerable due to the fractures and deformity. The

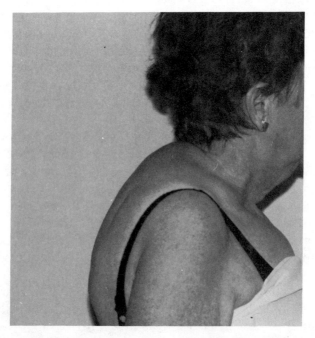

Figure 40. Photograph of a woman showing a dowager's hump.

pain problem may be relieved only by strong medicine. The combination of constant pain, deformity, and pain medicine may lead to discouragement and depression that may interfere with treatment. A person may give up and feel that nothing will ever help.

On the other hand, some people gradually develop a stooped posture over many years with very little pain. Except for the change in the shape of the back and loss of height, osteoporosis patients may be quite comfortable.

Treatment for Stage 4 is outlined in Chapter Five. Even though your grandmother may be in Stage 4 of osteoporosis, the treatment is still useful. These people know that they cannot return to the way they were many years earlier. But it is reasonable to have a goal of improvement in pain and mobility—improvement enough so that they may get around and do most of their desired daily activities in reasonable comfort. The way to attain this goal is to follow the guidelines for treatment. In these guidelines, the exercise program is very important. The exercises for the back strengthen the muscles of the back and improve flexibility, making the back more limber. This exercise program needs to be supervised, especially at first, to be sure the patient does the exercises properly and safely. We regularly see improvement if the program is followed. The stooped posture may persist, but the degeneration of the bones may be slowed or even stopped.

Encouragement is important. Osteoporosis patients often have other medical problems that need treatment as well. Depression may become worse if pain and limitation of activity continue. We occasionally see patients with severe depression who talk of suicide because of the constant pain, limitation, and discouragement over their future. These people must be convinced that improvement is possible so that they are able to begin the proper treatment. It truly is never too late to treat osteoporosis and try to prevent future fractures and limitation.

Q: A 63-year-old man asks, "I recently had a severe fracture of my ankle while getting off the subway. I slipped on some ice and my ankle just gave way. I am having a difficult time healing and I am still in a lot of pain after 3 months. Could osteoporosis be my problem?"

Men are also at risk for osteoporosis. This is often overlooked since menopause in women seems to be such an important cause of osteoporosis. In men, the disease is usually first discovered at a later age than in women, and may not cause fractures until age 70. If risk factors are present, however, it can happen much earlier. It is not possible to tell from your question whether you have osteoporosis. If the fall was not serious but the fracture was severe, it raises the possibility of osteoporosis which may have allowed the fracture due to less than normal bone strength.

Some risk factors which may contribute to osteoporosis in men include smoking and medical problems such as emphysema and chronic bronchitis. Heavy alcohol intake also increases the risk of osteoporosis. Some researchers have found osteoporosis and fractures in the spines of men who are heavy alcohol drinkers in their 30s and 40s.

In your case, it is important to be sure that you have no other serious medical problems. Some uncommon or rare diseases can cause osteoporosis or fractures and need specific treatment. Bone density tests can tell if osteoporosis is present and allow treatment to begin.

The healing process is not usually affected in osteoporosis. Fractures generally heal with treatment unless other problems delay healing.

Q: A 42-year-old woman asks, "I hate to exercise. The thought of long walks or playing tennis doesn't appeal to me. Is there something else that I can do to help myself?"

You are an honest person! Many of us do not have an exercise program. Many of those who do have an exercise program do not follow it regularly. Although lack of a regular program is an important risk factor in osteoporosis, it is only one of many risk factors.

It is best to try to include some level of exercise in your activity. We usually recommend 30 to 40 minutes of weight-bearing exercise at least three or four times weekly. This might include walking, running, or other activities. If you do not have the time and do not have the facilities, such as a gymnasium or health club, all is not lost. Think about your daily activities. You may be able to incorporate a reasonable amount of exercise in your daily routine. For instance, do you have stairs at your work or home? Walking and stair climbing at work certainly would count as weight-bearing activity. Perhaps you might be able to arrange your activity at work or home to include stairs or periods of walking. Use stairs instead of the elevator or escalator. Walk some shorter distances instead of driving. These are adequate weight-bearing exercises if done for the proper amount of time each week.

Weight-bearing exercise is important for two reasons. First, it turns out to be one of the strongest natural stimulations for bone formation. Also, weight-bearing exercises are easy and inexpensive to accomplish through such simple everyday activities as walking.

You should remember that even a brief exercise program is better than none at all. You should continue whatever portion of the program you can accomplish.

Lack of an exercise program is only one of the many risk factors attributed to the disease osteoporosis. You are also over age 40 which raises the risk of osteoporosis. If the exercise program is less than optimal then plans must be made to improve. If you have reached the best practical program for your schedule and time in life then you know that you are minimizing this risk factor as much as possible. Be careful to remove other risk factors to prevent osteoporosis.

Q: A 40-year-old woman asks, "I am 15 pounds overweight and osteoporosis does not run in my family. Should I really be so concerned?"

First, you must realize that you still have two risk factors for osteoporosis, i.e., you are over 40 years old and you are a female. These risk factors alone would not be alarming, although it should make you more careful of other risk factors. Our knowledge of the causes of osteoporosis does not allow us to tell how important one or two individual risk factors are for each person. There are probably certain risk factors which turn out to be more important in one person than another. The problem is that by the time we can understand which is the most important risk factor in each person, it is usually too late to do much prevention. Therefore, until we have a better knowledge of osteoporosis from researchers, we recommend removal of as many risk factors as possible. The fewer risk factors, the less likely it is you may develop osteoporosis. We also recommend following the other steps given to decrease the risk of osteoporosis.

Being 15 pounds overweight removes the risk factor of being underweight for your height. However, if other risk factors such as low calcium in the diet or early menopause are present, then the risk certainly increases.

Q: A 40-year-old mother asks, "My teenage daughter is a long distance runner. She has had several fractures which have kept her out of important races. She has had many tests and has been told by our physician that she should decrease her running. She still wants to enter the Olympic competition. Isn't there something she can do?"

This problem has become more apparent in young female athletes over recent years. It seems to be most common in runners. These athletes develop fractures in the bones of the feet. Many times the problem is caused by a form of osteoporosis. With vigorous training, especially long-distance running, menstrual periods may change or stop. The hormonal changes which cause this also cause osteoporosis because of lower levels of estrogen. With continued strenuous training, fractures may occur, especially in the lower legs and feet. It is important, of course, that other causes of bone weakness are considered by your physician.

There is no easy solution for your daughter's case. Athletes like her are highly motivated and well-trained. Many have reached high levels of competition because of their efforts. These women could decrease or stop training altogether, but that is not usually an acceptable solution to the athlete. Other possible ways to treat osteoporosis include brief periods of reduced activity and the use of calcium and estrogen. However, the decision of a method of treatment depends on each specific situation. This decision should be made with her physician to be sure of the best possible treatment for continued safe training.

Q: A 55-year-old woman asks, "I recently developed severe back pain and was found to have osteoporosis with a fracture in one of the vertebral bodies in the lower back. I also passed a kidney stone one year ago. Should I take calcium or should I avoid it since I had the kidney stone?"

You do have osteoporosis and fit into Stage 3, osteoporosis with fractures. You should see your physician to be sure no other causes of the osteoporosis are present. You should then begin to remove any risk factors possible which would help to minimize your osteoporosis. You should also consider those suggestions outlined in Chapter Five.

Calcium should probably not be given in your situation. It is true that taking calcium may increase the chances of kidney stones. In this case, you will need to talk to your physician who can help you decide if the benefits of calcium are worth the risks. Tests of the urine and blood may help in this decision.

Whether calcium is recommended or not, a decision needs to be made about the use of other treatments for osteoporosis since you had a fracture. Since each person is different and situations like this can be complicated, it is very important to follow the advice and guidance of your physician.

Q: *A 72-year-old man asks, "My physician has recommended that I have tests done to determine the degree of osteoporosis I have. I have had several fractures and have quite a bit of pain. But I am nervous about X-rays. Aren't they risky?"*

If the fractures are from osteoporosis, you would be in Stage 3, osteoporosis with fractures, or Stage 4, osteoporosis with deformities and chronic pain. It is never too late to begin treatment to try to decrease future fractures. The next fracture could be more serious, such as a hip fracture.

Some disturbing statistics show that when hip fractures occur in older people, up to 20 percent may stay in a nursing home or other facility for up to one year, 20 percent do not walk the first year, and up to 50 percent do not regain the ability to walk as well as they did before the hip fracture. Because of the other medical problems common in people of this age group, up to 20 percent may die within the first year.

These statistics make it very worthwhile to try to prevent future fractures. The treatment is usually simple to follow and can be reasonable in cost. Faced with the nation's bill for the cost of hip fractures today, the cost of prevention appears very reasonable.

Your concern about X-rays and radiation is understandable. Fortunately, you can be reassured that the methods involved in most osteoporosis screening tests used today are very safe. The exposure to radiation in dual energy X-ray bone density tests is minimal and considered to be quite acceptable. Of course, it is always good to avoid any unnecessary radiation or X-rays.

The value of a test for osteoporosis in your case would be to allow your physician to have some idea of the severity of your problem. It would also allow some measure of how effective your treatment is. If the test is repeated in the future after a period of treatment (such as one year), it may be possible to add other medications if progression of osteoporosis is shown.

Another reason the physician may want to have the osteoporosis testing performed would be to help in decisions about medication. Some medicines used in the treatment of Stage 3 and Stage 4 osteoporosis have potential side effects. If tests show very severe osteoporosis then it may help the physician choose from the available medications. Even if the osteoporosis testing is not done you should begin immediate treatment.

SUMMARY

1. Communication with your physician is vital in the treatment of osteoporosis.
2. People should look carefully at the risk factors for osteoporosis and evaluate their lives to see if increased risk is present.
3. Other diseases and the treatments for these diseases often increase the risk of developing osteoporosis.
4. The stages of osteoporosis are clearly indicated. People should define their stage according to age and other factors, and take control using steps for prevention and treatment.
5. It is never too early to be concerned with taking care of the body's health. Awareness of osteoporosis, the risk factors, prevention, management, and treatment are the keys to well-being.
6. With newer tests of bone density, osteoporosis can be detected early before fractures happen. Treatment works to prevent fractures, increases in health care costs, and disability in the future.

CHAPTER ELEVEN

Traveling with Osteoporosis Pain

We regularly see people with osteoporosis who think that they can no longer be active and travel. These patients have had a fracture in the spine, hip, or other area, and worry that many activities, especially travel, may be dangerous. For example, a 70-year-old woman we saw canceled a trip to Israel to see her new granddaughter. She had great fear of injury or fracture. Another 64-year-old woman told of canceling a flight across the country to her only grandson's wedding because of fear of hip fracture.

What is the answer? Do these persons with osteoporosis stop the extra activities? What is the risk involved with travel?

Discovering the diagnosis of osteoporosis by itself does not mean you must limit activities. In fact, as discussed in Chapter Seven, exercise is an important part of the prevention and treatment of osteoporosis. Walking is important as a strong natural stimulator of bone formation.

If you have a fracture from osteoporosis, then, of course, the fracture needs proper treatment. Your orthopedic surgeon will tell you when it is safe to resume usual activities. Remember, in osteoporosis the bones are thinner and may break more easily, but the fracture will heal with treatment. Your job is to prevent the *next* fracture. The ways to do this are outlined in Chapter Four.

Travel is an important way to maintain independence, increase your sense of well-being, and continue learning. Travel also helps you to stay active.

With osteoporosis, there is no limit where you can travel, within the country or internationally. The majority of international travelers are over 50 years old. This is because this group of people often has the time and financial means needed for longer trips. This age group also includes those people most likely to be affected by osteoporosis.

Plan Ahead

There are some simple steps you can take to make traveling easier. First, plan before you leave. Ask a travel agent to help you arrange a trip to a destination that fits your needs. For example, do you want a relaxing time at a beach, a resort, or a visit to a busy city like London? Try to match your location to the level of activity at which you feel most comfortable.

Pack Light

Pack only what you will need. Try not to be caught in an airport, at your hotel, or on a tour bus with several heavy pieces of luggage. Carrying heavy luggage can cause pain and fatigue that can affect your entire trip. Remember: You may not always have someone available to carry luggage.

One suggestion is to pack one or two small bags that you can carry on your shoulder. Assemble the clothes you plan to take on the trip, then take only half of them! You will find that you will do very well even if it means washing out some pieces of clothing in your hotel room occasionally. You'll enjoy the freedom from luggage more than you'll miss the extra clothes. Try to remember that you probably won't be invited on the spur of the moment to visit royalty—it is not necessary to take clothes for every possible event! Try to limit your bags to no more than 10 to 25 pounds total weight. You'll be glad you planned ahead.

Ask for Help with Luggage

Your travel agent can also help you travel at nonpeak hours. This will allow you to be sure that there is help available with baggage. With help, you can avoid lifting luggage, which can cause more back pain. Also, you can request a ride in a cart to avoid long walks in airports, which can often cause pain and make you tired. If you travel at busy times you may find it harder to find this help in an airport.

Fly Nonstop, If Possible

Try to arrange your flights so that they are nonstop, when possible. This will mean less changing of planes, less carrying of luggage, less standing, walking, and sitting in airports, and fewer chances for one of the flights to be delayed or canceled. All of these situations can cause more tiredness, more pain, and will take a toll on your travel enjoyment.

Take Extra Medications

Before your leave, check with your doctor to be sure that you have a supply of your medicines. You may have trouble finding the correct medicine at your destination, or you may have to spend part of your time finding a store with the proper medicine. Include a medicine to control the pain just in case it becomes worse while you travel.

Leave Space for Your Comfort

When you board your flight, don't hesitate to ask someone to help you put your carry-on luggage in the overhead storage. This will prevent the strain of lifting. It will also leave more space open for your feet and legs. This space will help prevent sitting in a cramped and uncomfortable position during travel.

Walk Up and Down the Aisle of the Plane

During travel in an airplane, you may find that the pain and stiffness become worse when you sit in one position for a while. You can help control this by walking up and down the aisle of the plane for 5 to 10 minutes each hour. This can help prevent stiffness and fatigue.

Stay on Your Exercise Program

Don't forget that exercises help keep you flexible, limber, and keep the muscles strong. This is especially helpful on a long flight. You can do many of the exercises in Chapter Seven while sitting in your airplane seat, especially those for the arms, legs, and neck. These exercises can help prevent stiffness, pain, and make you less tired when you arrive at your destination.

Choose a Hotel That Fits Your Needs

Try to choose a hotel that fits your needs. Many hotels now have heated swimming pools or whirlpools that you can use when you travel. Remember, it is important to continue your exercise program twice daily while you travel. It may not be as easy as at home, and it will often be inconvenient, but it is necessary to remain as flexible and strong as you were when you started.

To make your stay more comfortable, many hotels now have ramps at entrances to make walking easier. You may want to choose a hotel that has some rooms available with grab bars in the bathroom, toilet, or other areas. Your travel agent can help you to make sure you match your needs to the right hotel.

Pace Your Schedule

While at your destination, plan your schedule so that you don't have to do everything in one day. Try to make the amount of sightseeing or business reasonable for the time available. If you are with a tour group, try to make it a group that understands the value of rest as well as sightseeing. If you become too tired, you might need to miss some portions of a tour to rest and recover, then resume full activities later. In other words, learn to pace your schedule of activities so that you don't wear out too early in the travel. If you do this, you'll find that you accomplish about the same amount, but you will not have to suffer more pain, stiffness, and fatigue.

Protect Your Back and Joints

Protect your back and joints while you travel. Try to avoid unnecessary stress and strain in these areas with a few easy steps. For example, in a bus, plane, or train, sit with your buttocks against the back of the seat and with your back held straight, not stooped over. There is less pressure on the spine if we sit upright in this position than if we sit slumped. If there is less pressure on the back, there will probably be less pain and stiffness.

Another simple way to protect your back and joints is to avoid carrying heavy bags. Pack light and get help when the bags are moved.

When you plan visits to museums or other sightseeing, try to avoid carrying heavy equipment, cameras, or other heavy bags. This takes a toll on your back and joints and can greatly add to tiredness long before the day is finished. If walking is too tiring or causes pain, don't hesitate to rent a wheelchair or cart. Then you won't miss the sights, and you can keep up with everyone else. But you will still be much more rested at the end of the day, and the quality of your evening will be much better.

There are many more examples of smart ways to travel so that you can get around and do all the things you wish but still not cause severe pain, stiffness, and fatigue. Try to think of specific ways as you travel that will allow you to do all the activities, but not waste stress and strain on your back and joints. These are the keys to successful travel with osteoporosis and other painful conditions.

SUMMARY

1. Travel is important for independence. The diagnosis of osteoporosis is no reason to give up opportunities for fun and learning.
2. Plan ahead. Try to fly nonstop if you can, and talk with your travel agent about flying during nonpeak hours so you can receive help with your luggage easily.
3. Pack light. The less luggage you take, the less stress and strain on your body.
4. Take extra medications. Some prescriptions and medications are difficult to find overseas, so it is best to be prepared for emergencies.
5. Pace yourself. Do not try to see the world in one day! Take frequent rests and realize you can sightsee the next day . . . if you are rested.
6. Exercise even when traveling. Walk up and down the aisle on the plane to loosen stiff joints. Follow the exercises in Chapter Seven twice a day, and take advantage of the hotel's amenities such as a whirlpool, heated pool, or spa.

Glossary

Antacid   One of the many medications or other products which neutralize acid.

Calcitonin   A hormone which may decrease the rate of bone removal, sometimes used in the treatment of osteoporosis.

Calcium   A chemical element important to the body in bone formation.

Chronic Bronchitis   Inflammation of the bronchial tubes which is long-lasting and often results in cough and shortness of breath.

Chronic Pain   Pain or discomfort which lasts a long time or returns; often resistant to treatment.

Compression Fracture of Spine   A fracture in one of the spinal vertebral bodies in which the usually rectangular appearance is shortened or squeezed to a smaller size.

Conjugated Equine Estrogen   One of the most common forms of estrogen used in estrogen treatment.

Cortisone   A medicine which has been used widely for treatment of many diseases. Today, derivatives are more commonly used, especially prednisone.

Density of Bone   The amount or mass of bone present in a certain volume of bone.

Diabetes Mellitus   A disease involving decreased or absent effect of insulin and abnormally high blood glucose.

Dowager's Hump   The prominence in the upper part of the back commonly seen in older women.

Dual Energy Photon Absorptiometry   A test which allows measurements of bone mass in the spine, hip, or other areas and therefore can estimate if there is osteoporosis present.

Emphysema   A lung disease which causes shortness of breath which involves enlargement of the air spaces and destruction of portions of the lung.

Endometrial Biopsy   A sample taken from the inner lining of the uterus.

Estrogen   One of the female sex hormones which is produced by the ovary and is important in bone formation in women.

Femur   The bone in the thigh extending from the knee to the hip joint.

Fluoride   A chemical element which is sometimes used to treat osteoporosis.

Fracture   A break in a bone.

Hyperthyroidism   A condition in which there is an excess of thyroid hormone in the body.

Hysterectomy   Removal of the uterus by surgery.

Lactose   A sugar in milk which must be digested by the body's enzymes.

Lumbar Spine   The lower portion of the spine, below the thoracic spine.

Menopause   The period in which the end of menstruation occurs in women, most commonly from ages 45–55, when estrogen production by the ovaries decreases or stops.

Moist Heat   Heat applied using water or other moisture such as shower, whirlpool, tub, wet towels, or other similar methods.

Myocardial Infarction   Damage or death to a portion of the heart muscle by loss of blood supply, commonly called a "heart attack."

Osteoporosis   A bone disease in which the density of the bone is decreased because of a decrease in the amount of bone tissue present.

Ovary   One of the female reproductive glands which produces the egg and female sex hormones among other actions.

Pelvis   The bones formed by the ring of bones which supports the spine.

Peptic Ulcer   An ulceration involving the lining of the stomach or adjacent duodenum.

Progesterone   One of the female sex hormones which, among other actions, helps to regulate the menstrual cycle.

Pulmonary Embolus   Movement of a blood clot from a vein to block a blood vessel in the lung.

Quantitative CT (Quantitative Computed Tomography)   A computer test which allows measurement of volumes of bone in the spine to estimate the bone density and therefore estimate if there is osteoporosis present.

Radius   The shorter of the two bones on the forearm and on the same side as the thumb.

Rheumatoid Arthritis   A form of arthritis (usually long-lasting) with joint pain, stiffness, and swelling in the joints which may involve the hands, wrists, shoulders, knees, hips, ankles, feet, and other joints.

Risk Factors   In osteoporosis, one of the conditions that increases the chance of present or future osteoporosis.

Thoracic Spine   The middle portion of the spine, above the lumbar spine and below the cervical spine.

Thrombophlebitis   Inflammation of a vein or veins which may also be associated with a blood clot in the vein.

Treatable   Able to be given medical or surgical care.

Ulna   The longer of the two bones on the forearm and on the same side as the 5th finger.

Uterus   The female organ in which the fetus develops, also called the womb.

Vertebra   One of the single bones of the spinal column.

Vitamin D   One of several nutrients needed by the body for the use of calcium in bone formation.

Wedge Compression Fracture   A compression fracture of a spinal vertebral body so that the bone has a wedge-shaped appearance.

Weight-Bearing Exercise   Activity which involves the force of the body's weight on the skeleton such as walking, running, climbing stairs, and other activities.

Index

148